This book was a gift from Elisabeth! in 1983

We Gave Birth Together

We Gave Birth Together

Color Photographs and Dialogue of the Work, the Joy, and the Emotions of Childbirth

Karen Michele

with Elisabeth Bing

Photographs by Karen Michele

WILLIAM MORROW AND COMPANY, INC.
New York   1983

Photographs and Dialogue Copyright © 1983 by Karen Michele
Foreword and Commentary Copyright © 1983 by Elisabeth Bing

All rights reserved. No part of this book may be
reproduced or utilized in any form or by any means, electronic
or mechanical, including photocopying, recording
or by any information storage and retrieval system, without
permission in writing from the Publisher. Inquiries
should be addressed to William Morrow and Company, Inc.,
105 Madison Avenue, New York, N.Y. 10016.

Library of Congress Cataloging in Publication Data

Michele, Karen.
We gave birth together.

1. Natural childbirth—Pictorial works.   I. Bing,
Elisabeth D.   II. Title.
RG661.M5   1983   618.4   83-8146
ISBN 0-688-02233-2

Printed in the United States of America

First Edition

1 2 3 4 5 6 7 8 9 10

BOOK DESIGN BY ELLEN LO GIUDICE

To the people in this book—
Ken, Ellen, Ryan, and Kris Nelson;
Paul, Pat, and Alison Saccento;
David McCune, Susan Watt, and Douglas McCune;
and Thomas, Nancy, Kate, and Eric O'Connor—
who shared their experiences
in hopes of bettering those of others

—KAREN MICHELE

·Foreword·

Before Karen Michele came to see me, I had been quite sure that everything worth saying about the whole field of Prepared Childbirth, or even childbirth in general, had been said. Bookstores are filled with good books on labor and delivery, personal experiences, prepartum preparation, postpartum coping, new parents, new babies, psychological changes in a couple's life due to childbearing; books, in fact, on every imaginable approach to and about childbirth.

Why a new book? When Karen Michele showed me her stunning photographs of four couples before, during, and right after giving birth, I knew then there was an impelling reason for this book. Suddenly there was a new approach and a new chemistry through the combination of beautiful photographs, lively quotes from the participants, and explanations of what was taking place just then. Here was a book that could show dramatically in picture and word the emotional impact of birth.

I am convinced that every expectant mother and father will be helped by this book. It tells of the teamwork between a man and a woman and their absolute concentration on the amazing and difficult job at hand. Above all, it shows a kind of childbirth that should be available to everybody everywhere, one that occurs in a nonthreatening and relaxed atmosphere.

The four births described took place at the Maternity Center in New York City, a birthing center with easy access to a hospital to which women with sudden and unforeseen complications can be transferred. It allows a birth to take place in homelike surroundings, and members of the family are made to feel welcome and to become part of the experience. It is one of the most ideal places in which to give birth, and is a model for many centers in the country as well as for hospitals that are willing to allow couples to experience birth safely and in genuinely comforting surroundings.

The serenity and deep emotion that these couples felt are evident in the beautiful pictures. I hope this book will be an inspiration to many who will then become advocates of a deeply felt experience and thus help make this kind of birth possible for all women and men.

—Elisabeth Bing

·Acknowledgments·

I would like to thank:

Stanley Mann, for making so much possible.

Marla Johnson, Beth Scharfman, Chris Madden, Janet Reinbrecht, Etan Merrick-Mora, Leslie Sanders Axelrod, Jill Fischer Conway, Ed Hospedale, Beverly Brown, and Amber Michele Brown Hospedale, my mother, and the Maternity Center for their support and enthusiasm.

Alison Brown, my editor, for expressing such faith in this book and helping me to get through the difficulties in its completion.

—Karen Michele

Introduction

My interest in childbirth began several years ago when my favorite teacher was expecting a baby. When I asked her which hospital she would be delivering in, she told me that she and her husband would be having their baby in a birthing center, with a midwife attending. I was quite surprised by this, as I had never heard of this option before. Three days after her birth, I saw Noella, a beautiful, healthy little girl. I became fascinated as Claudette described the incredible experience of her daughter's birth, and I wanted to find out more about childbirth.

I began looking in bookstores and libraries for photographs that would show me what childbirth really looked like. But at best, all I could find were black-and-white photographs, often out of focus, in which I could barely distinguish the baby's head from all the sterile drapes. Even worse, these photographs failed to show what the parents were feeling.

I wondered what it was that was so mysterious about childbirth that made it almost unphotographable. It seemed as if film simply could not respond to the intensity of the situation. As a professional photographer, I knew that this could not be the case. It was then that I decided that one way or another, I was going to photograph the work, the joy, and the emotions of childbirth.

Last year, I met Ken and Ellen Nelson at a childbirth preparation class at the Maternity Center in New York. I explained to them that I was interested in photographing a birth from the emotional aspect rather than from a textbook one. We talked about some of our feelings about birth, and agreed that it should be very loving and intimate. Only after we had established a warm and trusting relationship did we make our commitment.

The last month of Ellen's pregnancy seemed like the longest month of my life. With each day that passed, I worried that she had given birth and that they had been unable to reach me in time. Finally, on a Sunday at 1:30 A.M., Ken called me to say that Ellen was in labor and that they were leaving for the Maternity Center.

I'll never forget the aura in the family room of the Maternity Center that night. There was excitement, yet a calm that can only be found when people are together, awaiting a miracle they know is just hours away.

When the baby was actually being born, I couldn't believe that I was lucky enough to be witnessing this incredible event. After Kris was born, I felt very close to the Nelsons as I shared in welcoming him. I was so happy when they asked me if I wanted to hold him. Taking Kris in my arms, I was filled with the wonder of all that had just happened. I looked at this tiny, beautiful boy, and I knew then that I was truly holding a miracle.

Several days later, I started showing the photographs of Kris's birth, and I was excited by the reactions. People of all ages were fascinated and moved by this photographic documentary. It was then that I decided to do this book.

I have spent the past year photographing childbirth at the Maternity Center. Together, the four couples in this book show a variety of experiences. The mothers range in age from their mid-twenties to their late thirties. Some are having their first baby, while others are enjoying the presence of their first child at the birth of their second baby. The labors and deliveries are relatively easy for some couples, longer and more difficult for others. But in all cases, the accompanying dialogue, taken from interviews I had with the parents, remains accurate and honest.

The couples chose to deliver at a birthing center where their individual needs would be respected. Because the mothers and fathers would be active participants in their babies' birth, their experiences would be a celebration of the love and trust they have for each other. It is my hope that once prospective parents can get this close to an actual birth, they will be better able to take an active role in choosing their method of childbirth.

Most of all, I want to share with you my sense of awe at the birth of a baby.

—KAREN MICHELE

·Labor and Delivery·

To better appreciate the emotions captured in these photographs, it helps to have a basic understanding of the physical progression of labor and delivery.

Some people say that one sign of approaching labor is having an excessive amount of energy the day before, such as wanting to clean the house thoroughly. It is better, however, to rely on more definite symptoms of real progression, like contractions becoming stronger and more frequent. There may be also the "bloody show," which is the loosening of the mucus plug that lodges in the cervix throughout the pregnancy. The plug is honeycombed with little blood vessels, so there may be a slight bleeding with its loss. If the membranes, or bag of waters, break, this is a sure sign to get in touch with the doctor or midwife.

Labor and delivery are understood more clearly when divided into three stages.

In the first stage of labor, uterine contractions cause the cervix, or mouth of the womb, to thin out and retract. This is called "effacement." At the same time, the contractions cause the upper muscles of the uterus to shorten, pulling the cervix open. This is called "dilation," which is generally measured in centimeters. Full dilation is at ten centimeters. Since the first stage is the longest part of labor, it helps to divide it further into three phases.

The first phase includes dilation to about three or four centimeters. Labor usually starts slowly. There is a long period when little happens. Contractions are irregular, and though they cause the cervix to efface, little progress is shown when the mother has her first examination. It can be quite disappointing to find that after hours of contractions, she may have dilated no more than one or two centimeters. It takes an average of eight to nine hours to dilate three or four centimeters; and while some women may take twenty-four hours, others may require only a few hours.

However, labor speeds up eventually, and once active labor starts, when contractions are likely to occur every two to three minutes, dilation progresses more rapidly. In this second phase, dilation will increase from about three to four centimeters to approximately seven or eight centimeters. On average, this process will take three to four hours. By the time the woman sees her doctor or midwife, she should be well advanced and dilating. She also should be using some relaxation and breathing techniques to help her stay in control of her contractions. Contractions are like ocean waves that she has to maneuver, staying on top of each wave as it comes along. It helps to change positions from sitting to standing to resting in bed. Walking around can help labor progress more rapidly.

Usually the most difficult part of labor is "transition," during which the cervix opens from about seven or eight centimeters to full dilation at ten centimeters. The contractions become even stronger, closer together, and more difficult to cope with. At this point, it will be hard for the mother to stay in control, and she will need a great deal of love and support from her partner. Fortunately, this is the shortest phase. It generally takes about an hour of intense concentration and work, after which the cervix has opened enough to allow the baby to pass through it into the birth canal. The delivery of the baby begins, which is the second stage of labor.

In the second stage, the middle and upper muscle fibers of the uterus contract to expel the baby slowly through the birth canal. During this period, the woman experiences a compelling urge to bear down and push the baby out. It takes approximately one and a half hours to push out a first baby. A second baby may require about half that time.

In the third stage of labor, after the umbilical cord is cut, the placenta or afterbirth becomes detached from the inner wall of the uterus. The uterus contracts again to help expel the placenta. Stage three takes just a few minutes.

ELLEN
· and ·
KEN

Ellen: I was about eight days past my due date by the time I went into labor, and feeling very anxious about it. Everyone was expecting the baby to be early, so the last week seemed eternal. On this particular day, Kenny and I had gone to a wedding. I was having such a great time that I wasn't quite as focused on waiting for the baby as usual. During the wedding, I wasn't aware of any signs of labor, but as soon as we got into the car and settled down for the drive home, I began having strong contractions. I figured the contractions would end when I got home. I didn't want to get too excited about being in labor, and then be disappointed. But by midnight the contractions were coming regularly. I looked at Kenny and said, "Come on, this is it!" He was pretty casual about things, and wanted to wait an hour to be sure.

Kenny: Ellen had been having Braxton-Hicks for days, so I wondered if this wasn't just more of the same. I thought waiting a bit would tell us whether or not she was really in labor.

Ellen: I waited the extra hour, practically staring at the clock the whole time. I knew I was in labor for sure, and said, "OK, the hour's up. We're going!" At this point, the contractions were six to seven minutes apart, and about forty-five seconds long. We called the midwife, Karen. She was great. "I think you are in labor," she said. "Since this is your second baby, I think it would be best for you to start in now." So we gathered up our things, woke our six-year-old son, Ryan, and set off.

Braxton-Hicks contractions

Toward the end of a pregnancy, the uterus already starts contracting at irregular intervals. This is like practicing for labor, and, although no dilation takes place as yet, the contractions often move the baby well into the pelvis. These contractions are called Braxton-Hicks contractions, named after an Englishman who first described them. It may be difficult occasionally for a woman to tell whether her contractions are the ones that cause the cervix to dilate, or those that are felt before labor begins.

Kenny: We arrived around two A.M. Ellen was marvelous, cracking jokes and talking calmly in between contractions. Ryan fell asleep on the couch, and I unpacked our things. By this time, Ellen was really in active labor. The contractions were coming every two to three minutes. Karen's examination revealed that she was approximately five centimeters dilated. At this point, I thought it would be much longer before the birth than it actually was. We all sat down and talked for a while.

Ellen: I was so happy here. I had just had a great time at a wedding, and now I was going to have a baby! I felt so lucky. How can anyone have so much fun in one day? I guess a lot of people don't exactly think of labor as being fun, but I like it. It's different from everything else, in that no one can do it for you. Having a baby is just the most incredible experience in life, and I knew that my delivery here was going to be very special.

It was so nice not having to be moved into a sterile setting. I mean, there I was, drinking my ginger ale and laughing with the people who'd been looking forward to sharing this birth with me. Everyone around me was as happy as can be, and I loved it!

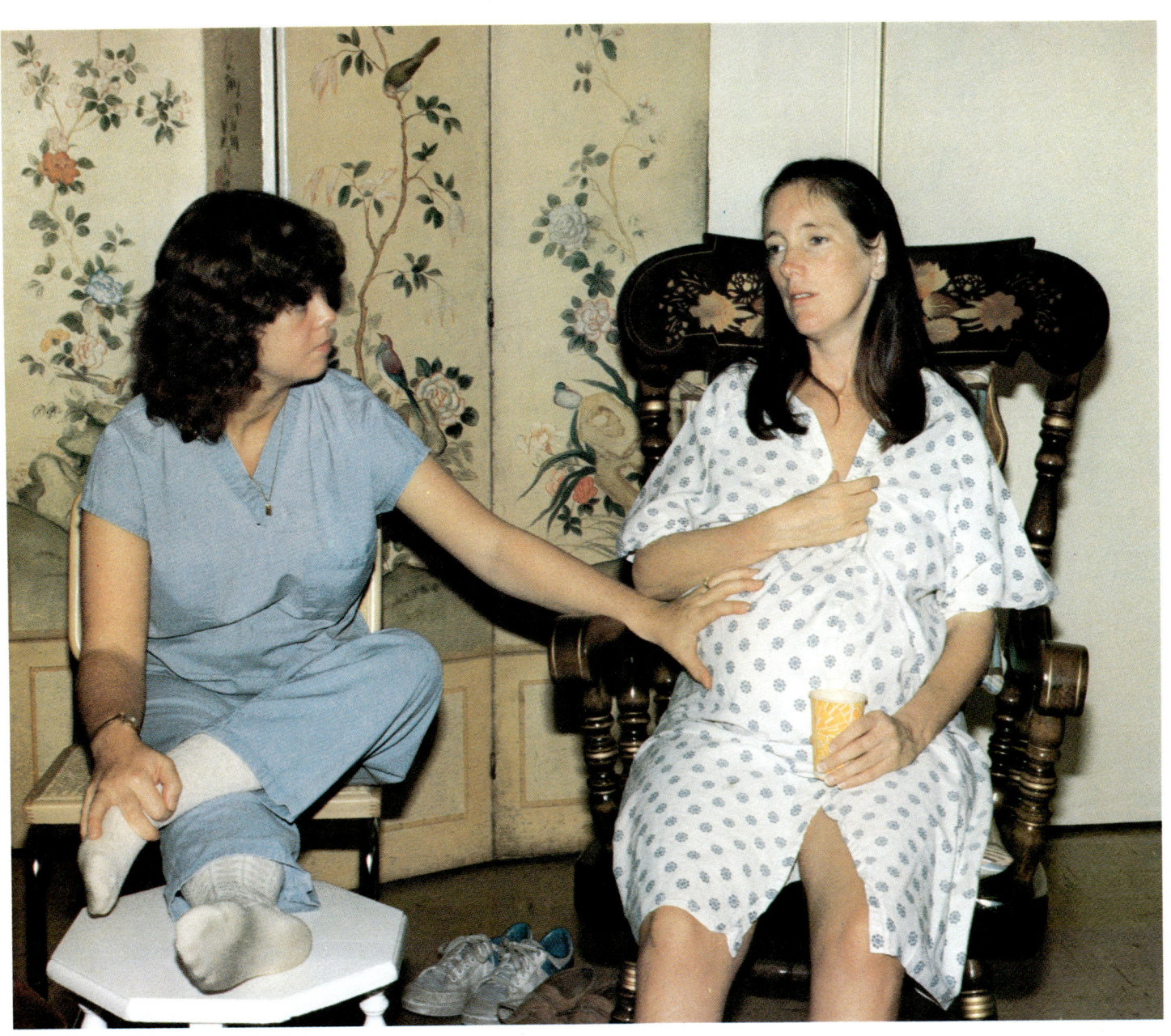

Ellen: Right from the start, I had a good feeling about our midwife, Karen. She respected my need to feel in charge of my labor. Before making decisions, she consulted with me, asking me how I felt and what I thought. Whenever something had to be done, she always explained why. She made sure that I always knew just what was happening. Her presence was always calming, and I felt that she considered my happiness and relaxation to be of paramount importance. Her touch was phenomenal. It was like a magnet that could draw all the tension out of my body. When I had a contraction, she would gently put her hand on my stomach. From this light touch, she could tell just how that contraction felt. I've never seen anyone more thorough, and yet so gentle. Even her exams during labor didn't bother me.

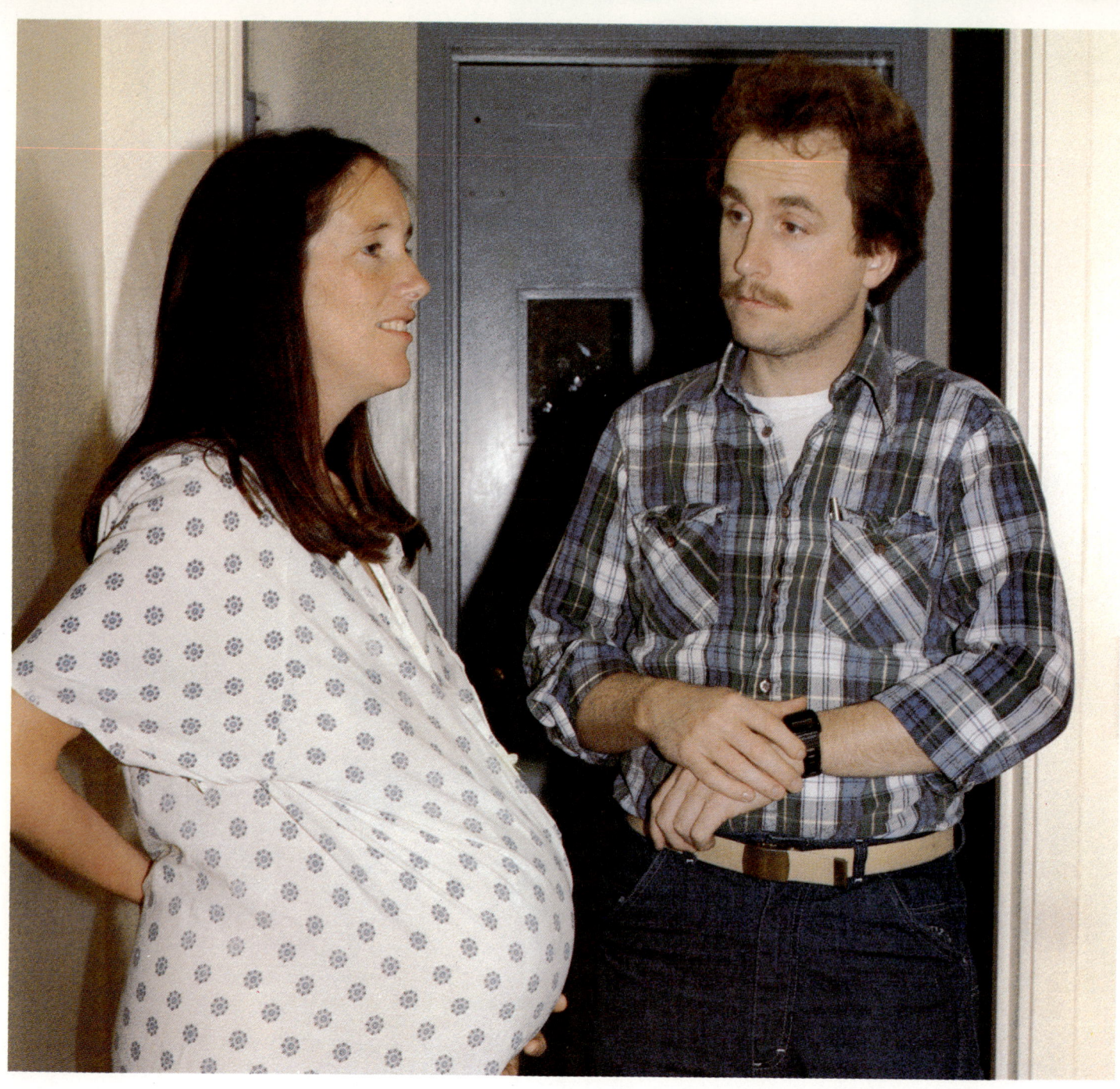

Kenny: During the time that Ellen was sitting still, the contractions slowed down quite a bit. In fact, they were barely coming at all. Karen noted that the contractions were much stronger and more consistent when Ellen was up and about. She suggested that Ellen take a walk around the building. We followed her advice, and the labor began to progress very quickly.

Ellen: Kenny was such a great help. Oh, he was so wonderful. I was feeling kind of lazy and just wanted to sit around. Kenny encouraged me to keep walking by making little jokes about the exciting sights in the hallway, and by reminding me that this was the best way to keep the labor moving.

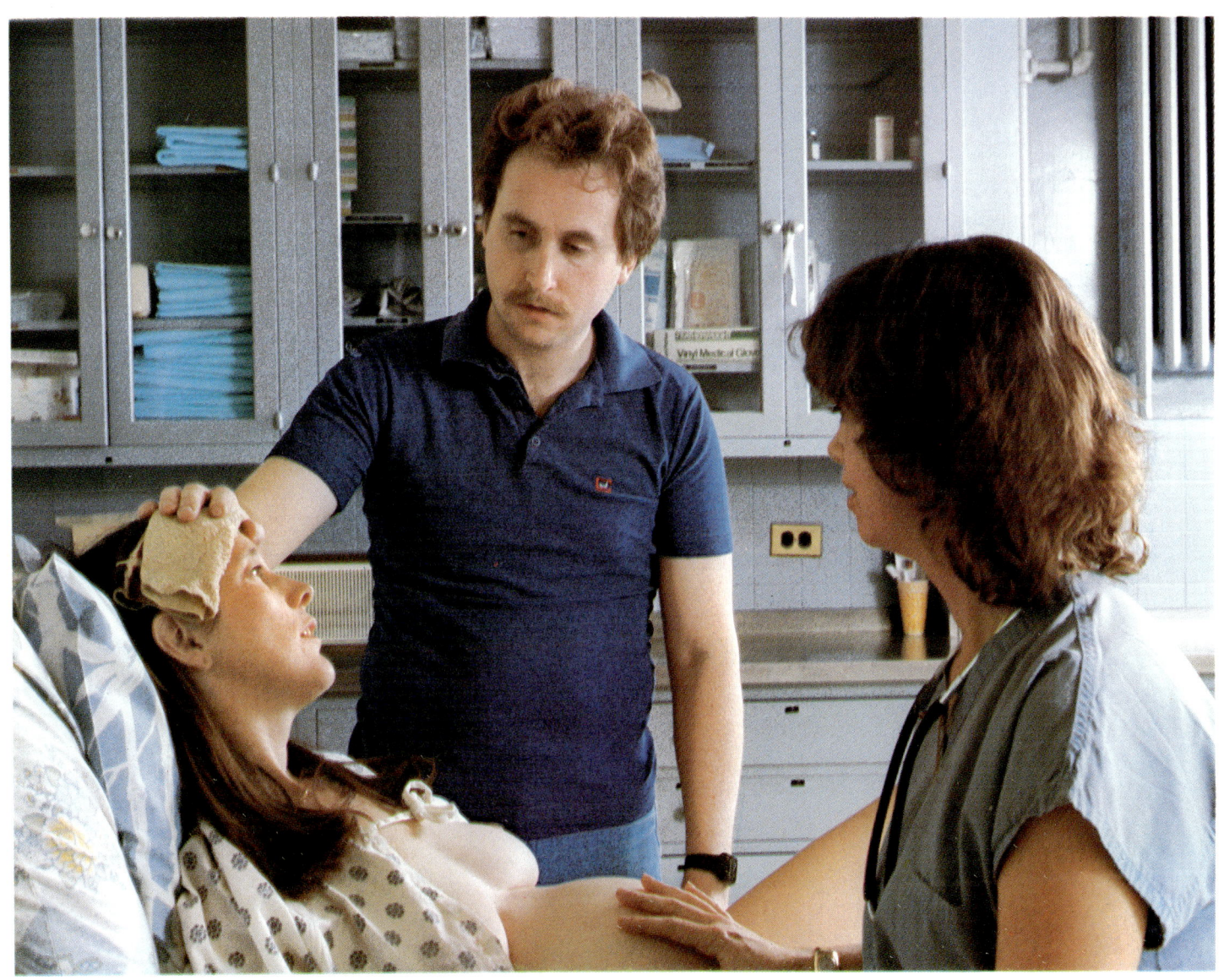

Kenny: In the beginning, I was maybe a little nervous. It was very different here than when Ellen gave birth to Ryan in a hospital. There, the nurses did everything, and I had to stay in the background. But I was sure I could handle things this time. Once Karen confirmed that everything was going smoothly, I felt excited to be as closely involved as I was. This was, after all, the birth of my child, and being able to share the experience with Ellen, and of course be helpful and reassuring to her, were very important to me.

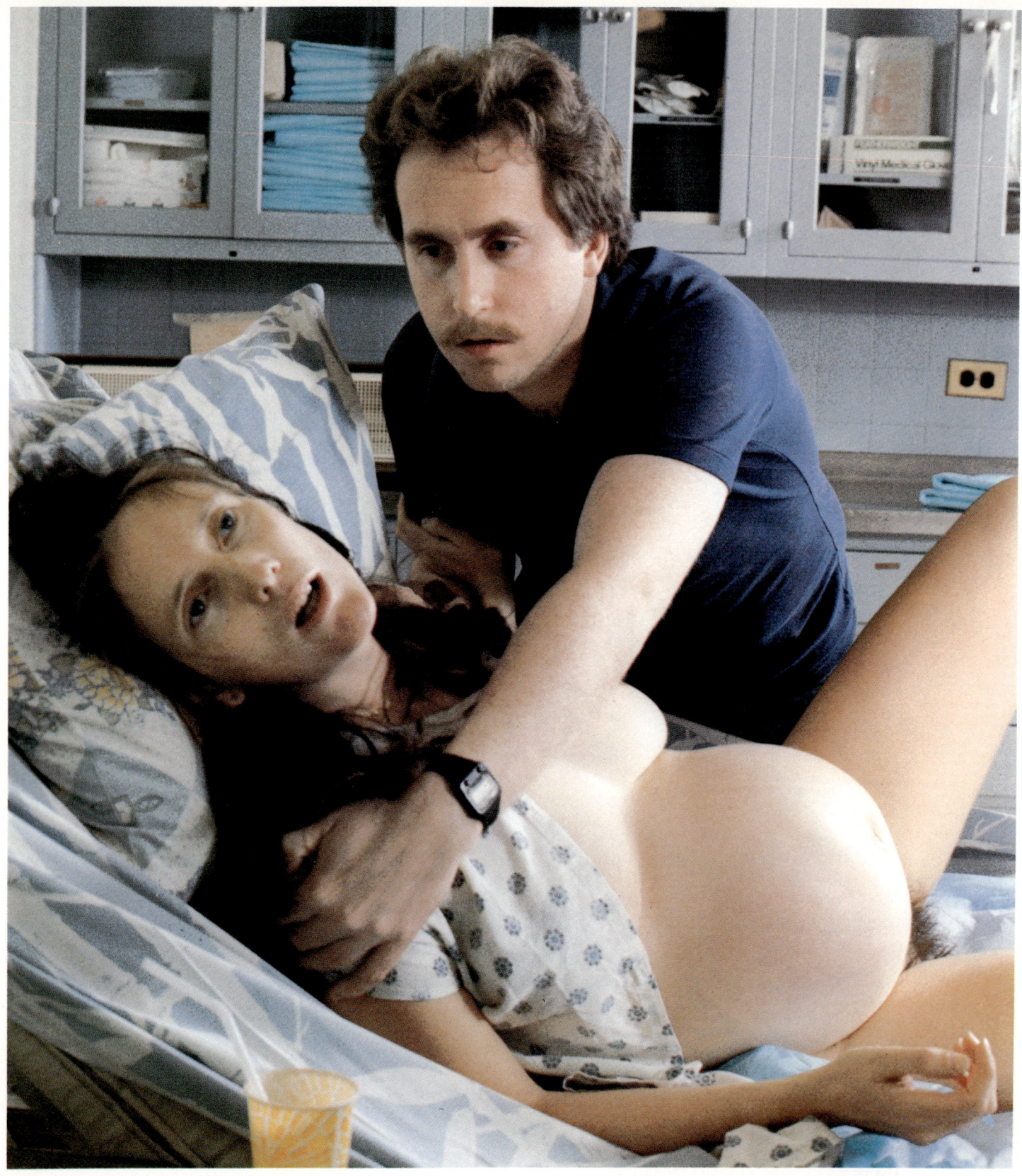

Kenny: Throughout transition, even when the contractions were difficult, Ellen remained in touch with me in some way. She was able to relax or at least follow my instructions when she needed a reminder. But this contraction was the strongest one of all. She lost her concentration, she wasn't doing her breathing, and she lost contact with me. She went completely limp, and it looked as if she might even fall off the bed. Immediately I grabbed her, made

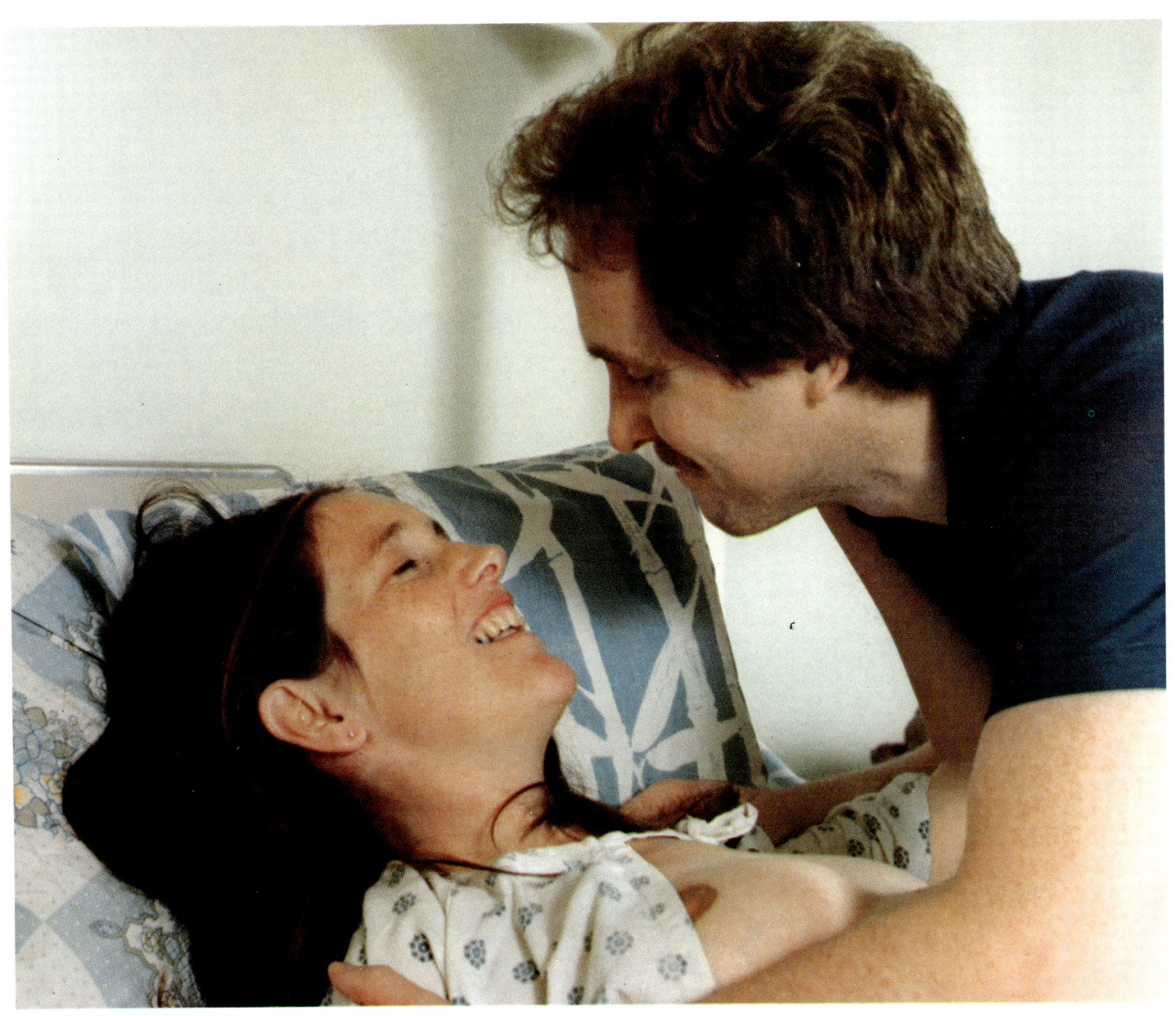

sure she saw me, and tried to bring her back. I told her that I knew the contractions were coming very hard and fast, but that she was doing very well and the baby would be here soon. She seemed relieved to see and hear me. It was as if for that moment, she'd forgotten that I was there with her. This contraction marked the end of transition, and she was now ready to start pushing.

Pushing
Being told one can push is very satisfying. The mother's whole body wants to expel the baby. She concentrates completely on helping her baby out into this world. But even now it is good to work gently and without too much force.

The pushing stage is like going two steps forward, then one step back. When the mother pushes, the baby moves down, but when the contraction is over, the baby slips back a little.

Ellen: I remember Kenny wanting to go and see if the baby's head was showing yet.

Kenny: She said, "Ken, don't leave me!" I told her that I wasn't going anywhere. She held out her hands and said, "I don't mean to take this away from you, but I need you right here!"

Ellen: It wasn't that I really needed him, I just wanted him. I don't think I've ever wanted to be as close to anyone as then. I figured he could still see the baby come out. He wasn't so far away that there would be a problem. But for that moment, I just wanted him to hold me.

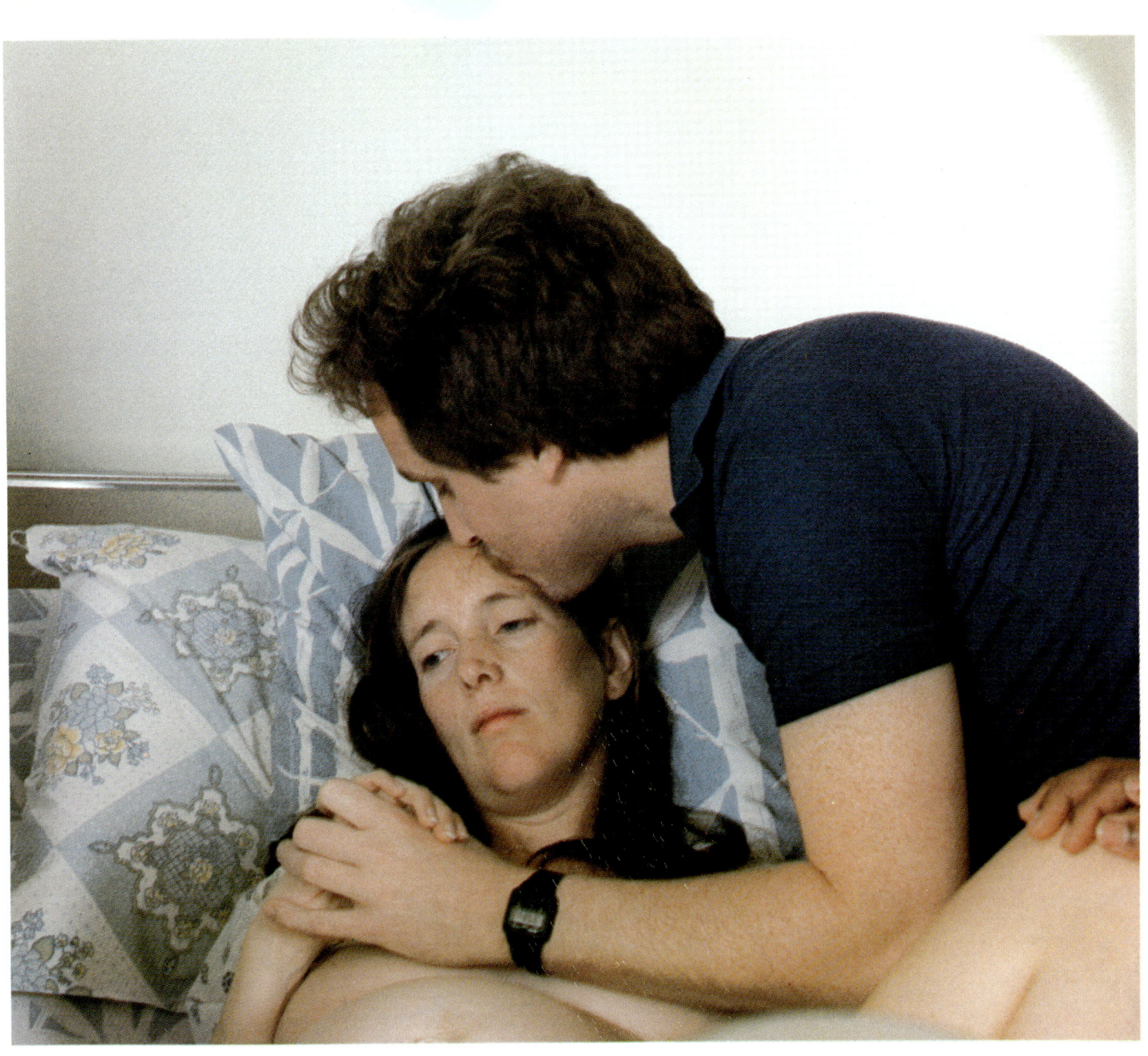

Ellen: Pushing was so difficult, mostly because I wasn't ready for it. I never thought I'd have to push that hard. I remember that the baby was very low down and was putting a lot of pressure on my rectum. I hated that and kept complaining, "It hurts!" I heard afterward that the pushing took only eighteen minutes, but at the time it seemed like hours. One thing that really kept me going was looking up at everybody and being able to see faces instead of surgical masks. They were smiling, and that was most encouraging.

Kenny: I was feeling very confident. Ellen and I were much more prepared this time than when Ryan was born, and Karen was terrific. As soon as I saw a little dark circle emerging, I knew it was the baby's head. I got even more excited, knowing that it would be just a matter of moments before we could see and hold our baby.

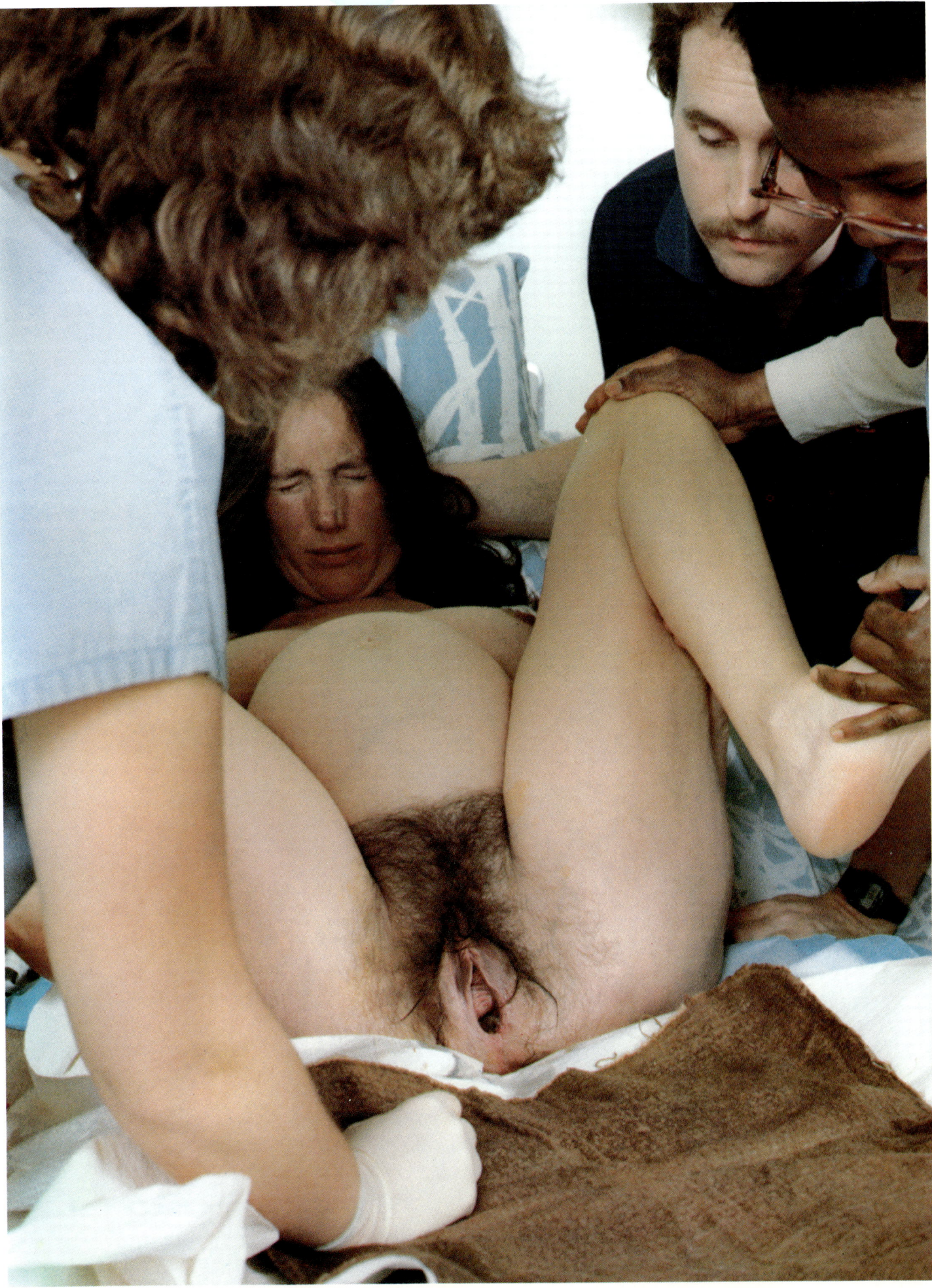

Ellen: In between contractions I had a brief moment when I first realized how naked I was. I remember thinking, "I'm completely naked! I should be upset or something, but I'm not. This feels great!" Everyone around me was so warm and caring that there was no reason for me to feel self-conscious.

It was so much nicer here than it was last time when I had to be covered up in sheets and gowns. The whole nonsense with the sterile drapes and the leggings made that birth experience seem more like a surgical procedure than a beautiful event.

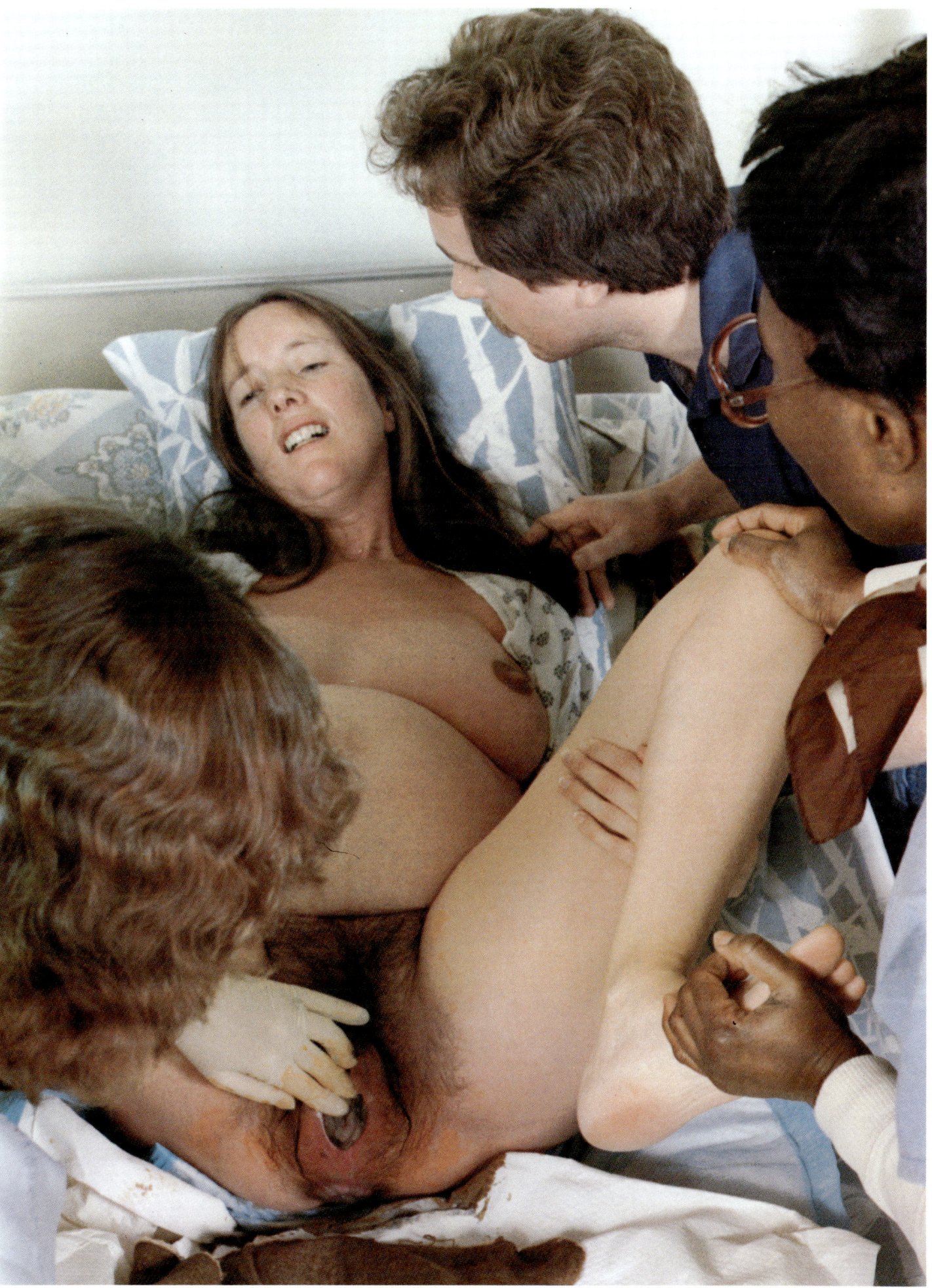

Ellen: I had told Karen that, if possible, I didn't want to have an episiotomy. I knew this might be difficult because for Ryan's birth, I had no choice and was given a routine episiotomy. Because of this, the skin would be weaker and more apt to tear. When the time came, Karen was very sweet and tried her best to stretch my perineum gently. But the baby's head was big, and there just didn't seem to be a large enough opening. As I was pushing with a contraction, I began to tear in the same place where the scar was. Karen said, "Listen, I'm sorry but I have to do an episiotomy. The perineum is not stretching enough for the baby, and you're beginning to tear." I knew she was right.

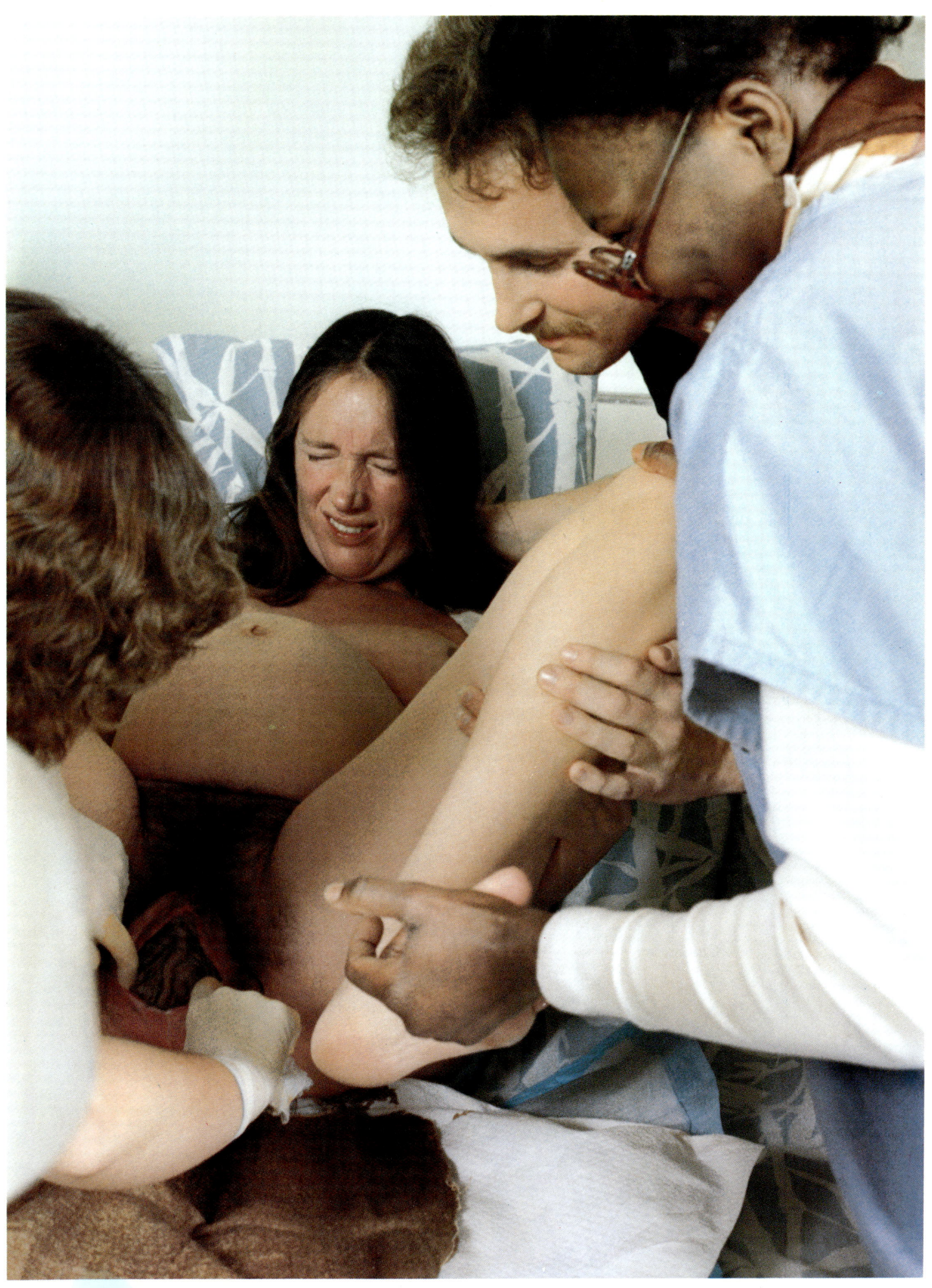

Ellen: When somebody says they're going to have to cut you, it's hard to keep calm. But I trusted Karen implicitly, and I knew that she would do the episiotomy with great care, making it only as large as necessary. She told me to blow if I had a contraction, so as not to push the baby's head toward the scissors. There was so much pressure from the baby's head that I hardly felt the cut.

Episiotomy

The episiotomy is a small surgical procedure that is frequently performed. It is an incision made in the perineum, the area between the vagina and the anus. The cut is made either in a straight line—the median cut—or slightly off to one side—the mediolateral cut.

Such an incision is not always made. It depends on several factors, including the size of the baby's head, the rotation of the head, the elasticity of the perineum, and the mother's ability to control her pushing. Above all, it depends on the midwife or doctor who is in charge of the delivery. Often this person can avoid the episiotomy by gently massaging the perineum, using oil or Castile soap. If, however, the tissues become white and overextended, and look as if they might tear, the doctor or midwife may prefer to perform the episiotomy. An incision may also be necessary when it becomes imperative to get the baby out as fast as possible.

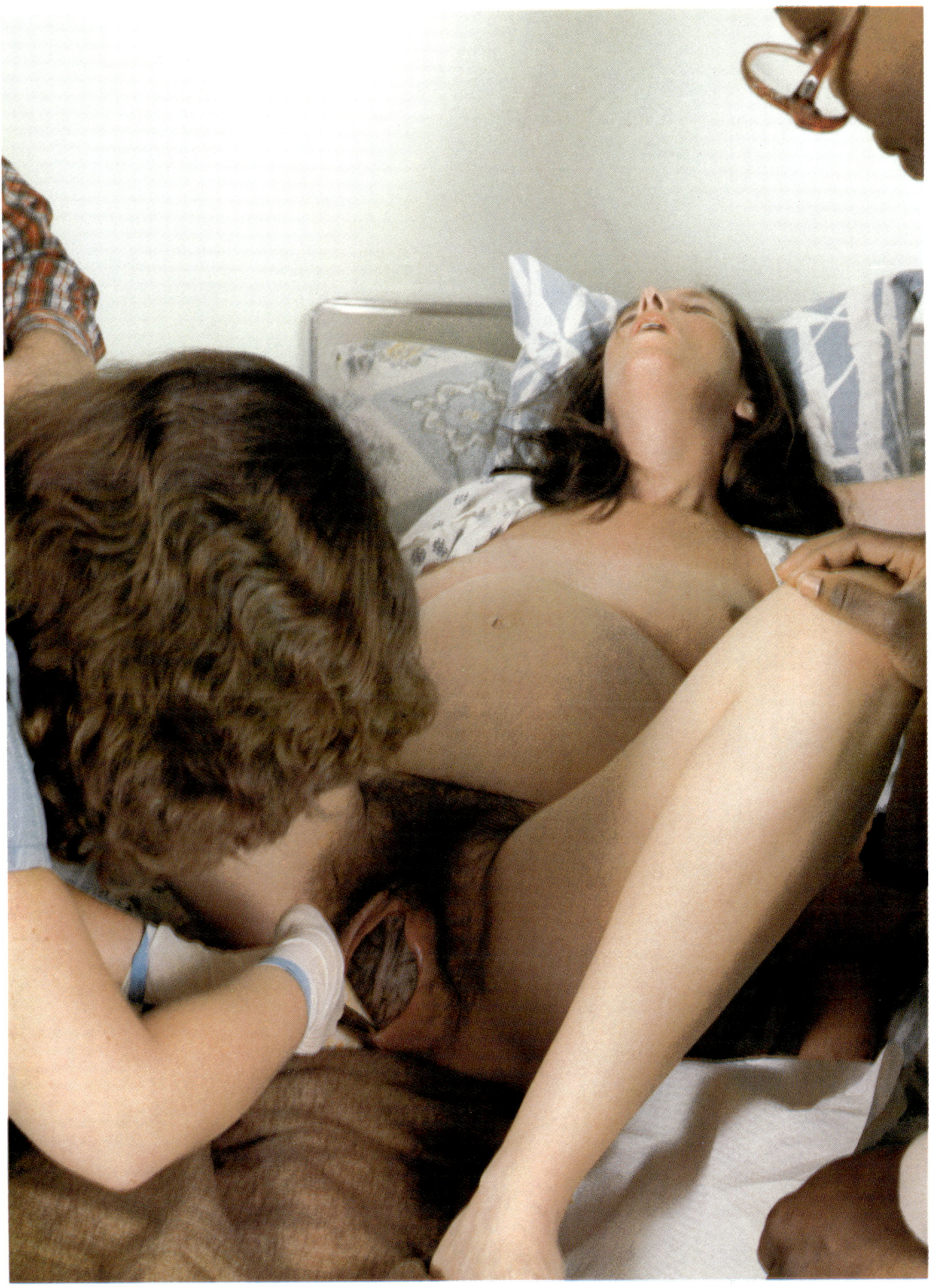

Ellen: I knew the episiotomy had made the opening large enough for the baby. Once its head was out, I didn't need to push anymore, so I just relaxed while Karen allowed the baby to rotate, and the rest of its body came out.

Rotation of the baby

Most babies start out by facing either one or the other of their mothers' hips. Then during the first stage of labor, the baby is slowly rotated so that it faces down toward its mother's spine. When the mother starts to push, the crown of the baby's head shows first at the exit of the vagina. As the crown stretches the outlet of the vagina, the baby's head emerges and faces straight into the world for a few seconds. But then the baby is in trouble, for it can't get its shoulders out squarely. Therefore, a second rotation occurs. This is called the "external rotation" because the head is already out when the baby turns again, usually toward the hip it faced at the start. The midwife or doctor supports the baby's head and gently helps the upper shoulder and arm out first. After the second shoulder and arm, the rest of the baby's body simply slips out.

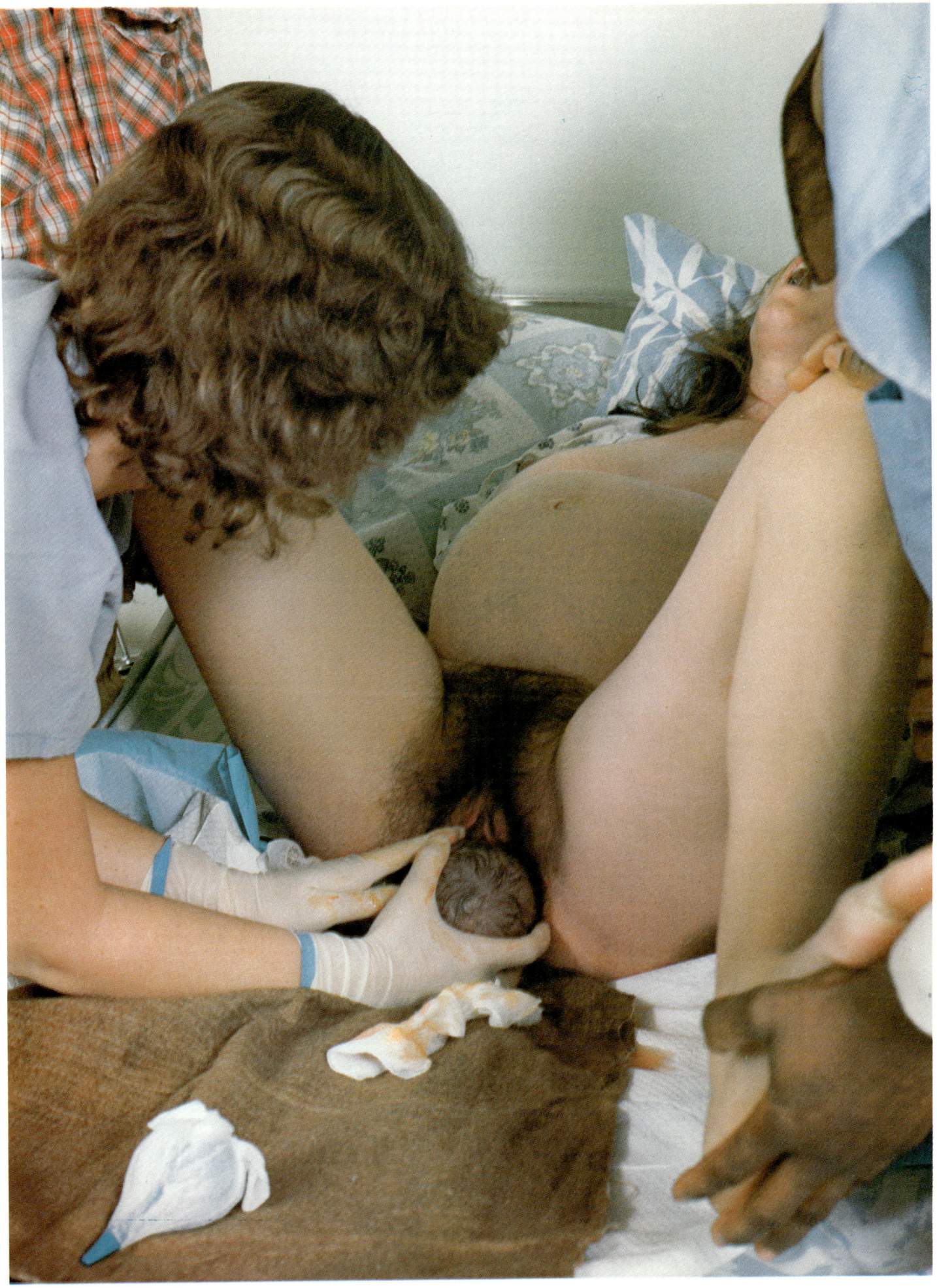

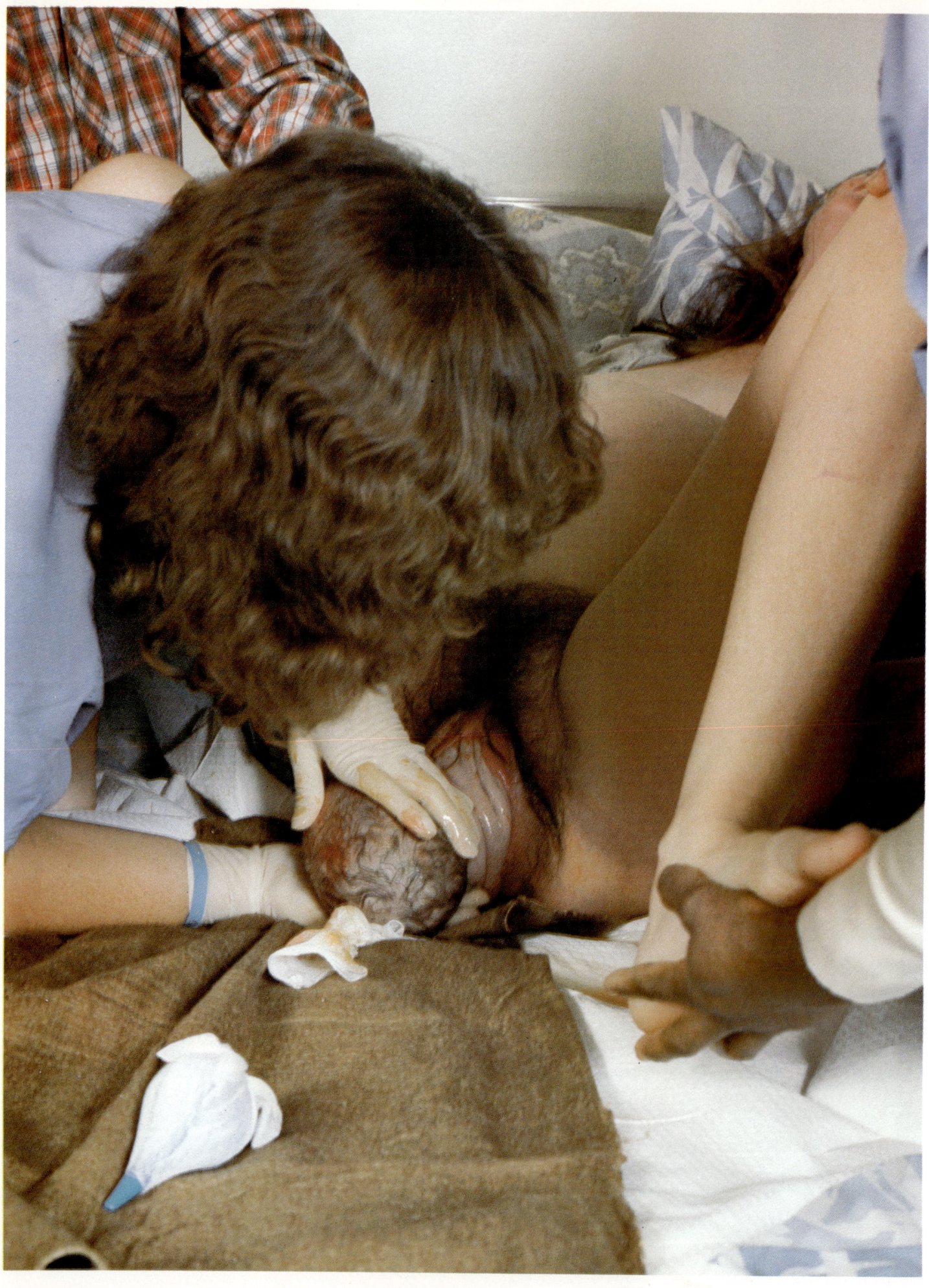

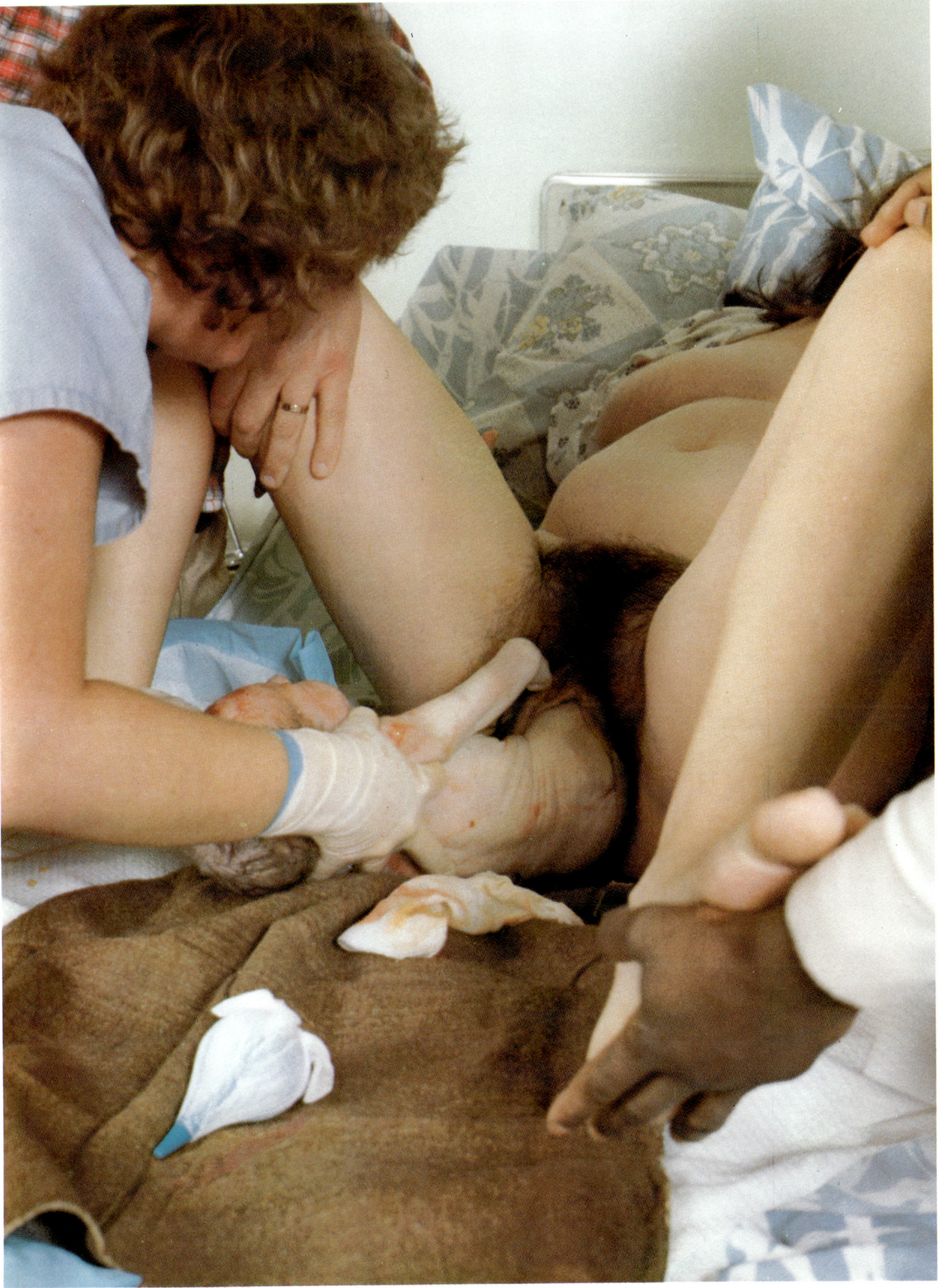

Kris has entered our world
This is Kris at birth. You can see the umbilical cord has not yet been clamped and cut. It leads to the placenta, which is still attached to the upper wall of the uterus. Kris is wet from the amniotic fluid that accompanied his exit from the womb. There is relatively little blood on his head and chest. It is his mother's blood; some of the small blood vessels in the cervix break during the baby's descent. If you look closely, you can see a little white creamy substance just under the baby's arm. This is called "vernix." Babies are born with it in varying amounts. It acts as a protective cream while the child lives in the womb.

The cord is light blue and is about three quarters of an inch thick. It is actually wound like a cord. Kris's genitals seem large, which is normal in a newborn.

Kris is a very healthy color. Most newborn babies' skin looks grayish blue, but turns pink very quickly. However, the hands and feet tend to stay blue for a while, which is due to comparatively poor blood circulation in the extremities.

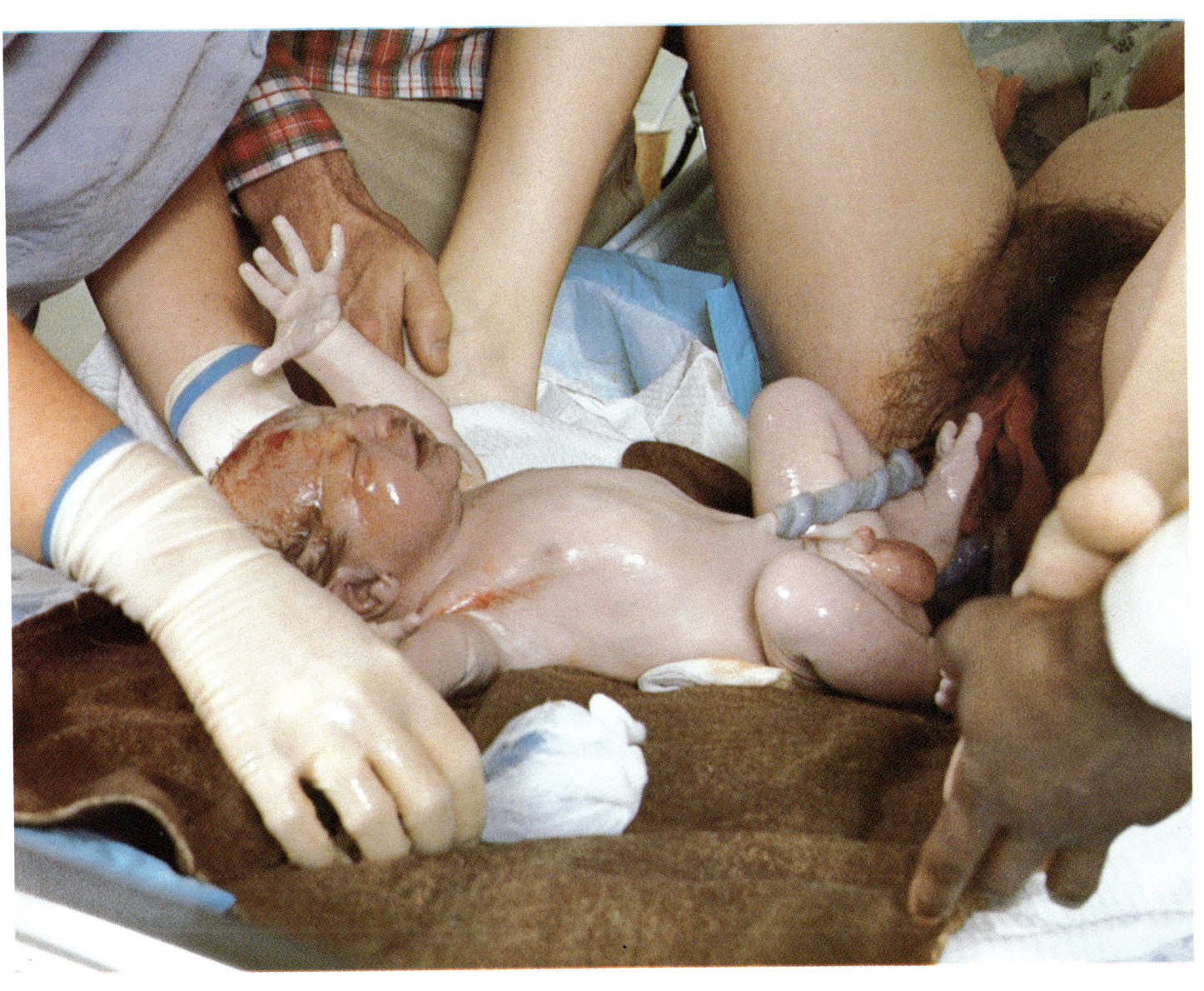

Ellen: I thought he was so beautiful! Karen left him right there on the bed with me so I could see everything that was happening to him.

Kenny: As soon as Kris was born, he lay there looking around with his eyes wide open. He was calm, and it was wonderful to see how well he was adjusting to his new environment. I was pleased that the umbilical cord wasn't cut right away. This gave him a chance to get used to depending on his own life-support systems. He remained attached to his mother for at least five minutes while Karen dried him off and aspirated his nose and mouth. By the time she clamped the cord, we could all see that he was breathing well and was a healthy pink color.

I was in such awe, watching the baby, that I was completely surprised when Karen handed me the scissors and asked me if I wanted to cut the cord. I felt happy to do this, knowing that he was ready to take the first step toward becoming his own person.

Cutting the umbilical cord
Once the baby is born and has started to breathe on its own, it is time to tie and clamp the umbilical cord. The midwife or doctor will wait until the cord has stopped pulsating, and then will tie the cord about an inch from the navel, clamping it about two inches farther away. Sometimes the father will be offered the scissors to cut the cord. This is a lovely act with all its implications of separating the new little life. The cutting does not hurt the baby, as there are no sensory nerves in the cord.

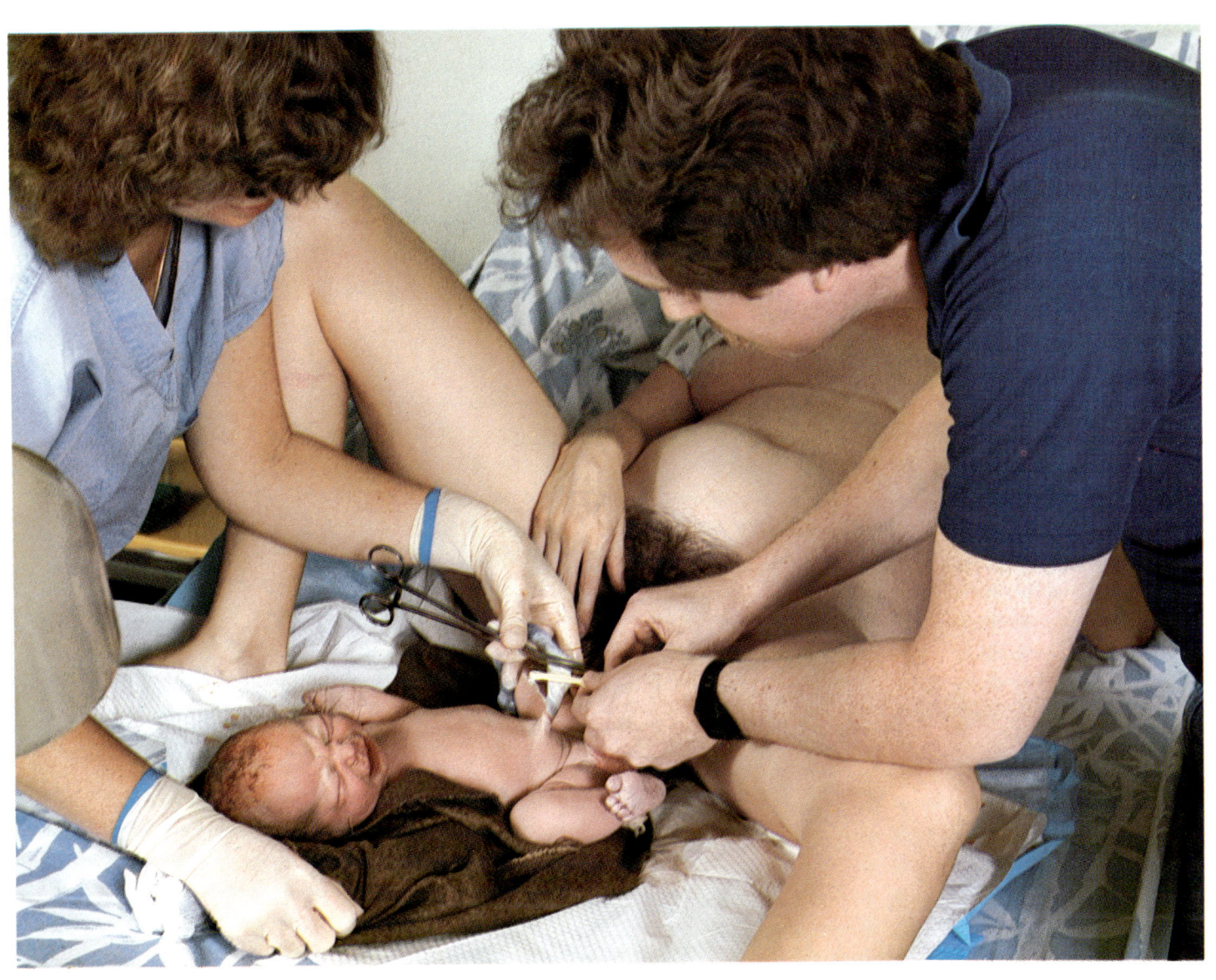

Ellen: I held Kris for a while, but then started having afterbirth pains. It was four-thirty in the morning, and I was just exhausted. I needed to lie still, and Kenny was happy to take the baby from me. I was glad that they had a chance to bond, and I loved watching them together.

Kenny: I felt very proud of my little son. From the second he was born, he was awake, alert, and eager to explore his new world. I was so happy that Kris was mine. I loved him immediately; not just because he was mine, but because I felt there was really something special between us. I spent most of the next few hours holding him, and he seemed to know that we belonged together.

Contractions after the baby is born
Once the baby is born and the placenta has been expelled, the uterus contracts again in order to decrease in size and return slowly to its normal nonpregnant state. This is called "involuting." The contractions that cause the uterus to shrink are often quite noticeable. If the baby is the mother's second or third child, she will be even more aware of these "afterbirth pains" because the uterus has been stretched before, and it will take longer to return to its nonpregnant size.

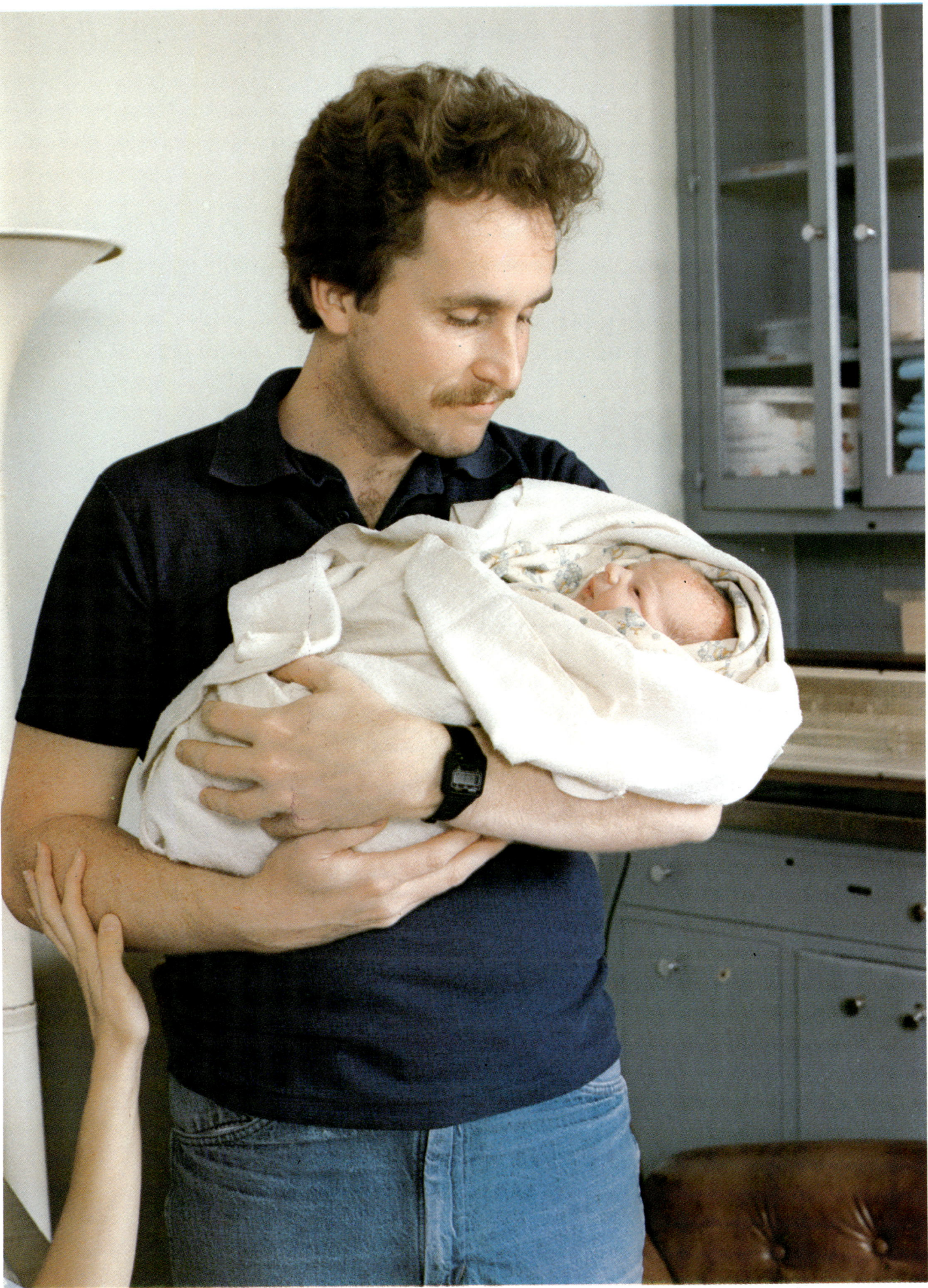

Ellen: We asked somebody to go wake Ryan and bring him in to us. I thought it was so great having him there. Nothing could have made this better than being able to have the most important people in my life there with me. Ryan is a better person, too, having had this experience. It didn't matter that he slept through the actual birth, as long as he knew that he could be there if he wanted to. It was good for Ryan to be able to see his parents so happy, and to understand how much this new little baby meant to all of us.

A parent can give so much to a child in material things, but telling Ryan that we wanted him to be with us meant much more to him. I think that he will always feel proud that he was a part of Kris's birth. When he grows up, he will remember it, and he will seek out the qualities in life that can be found only in family and friends.

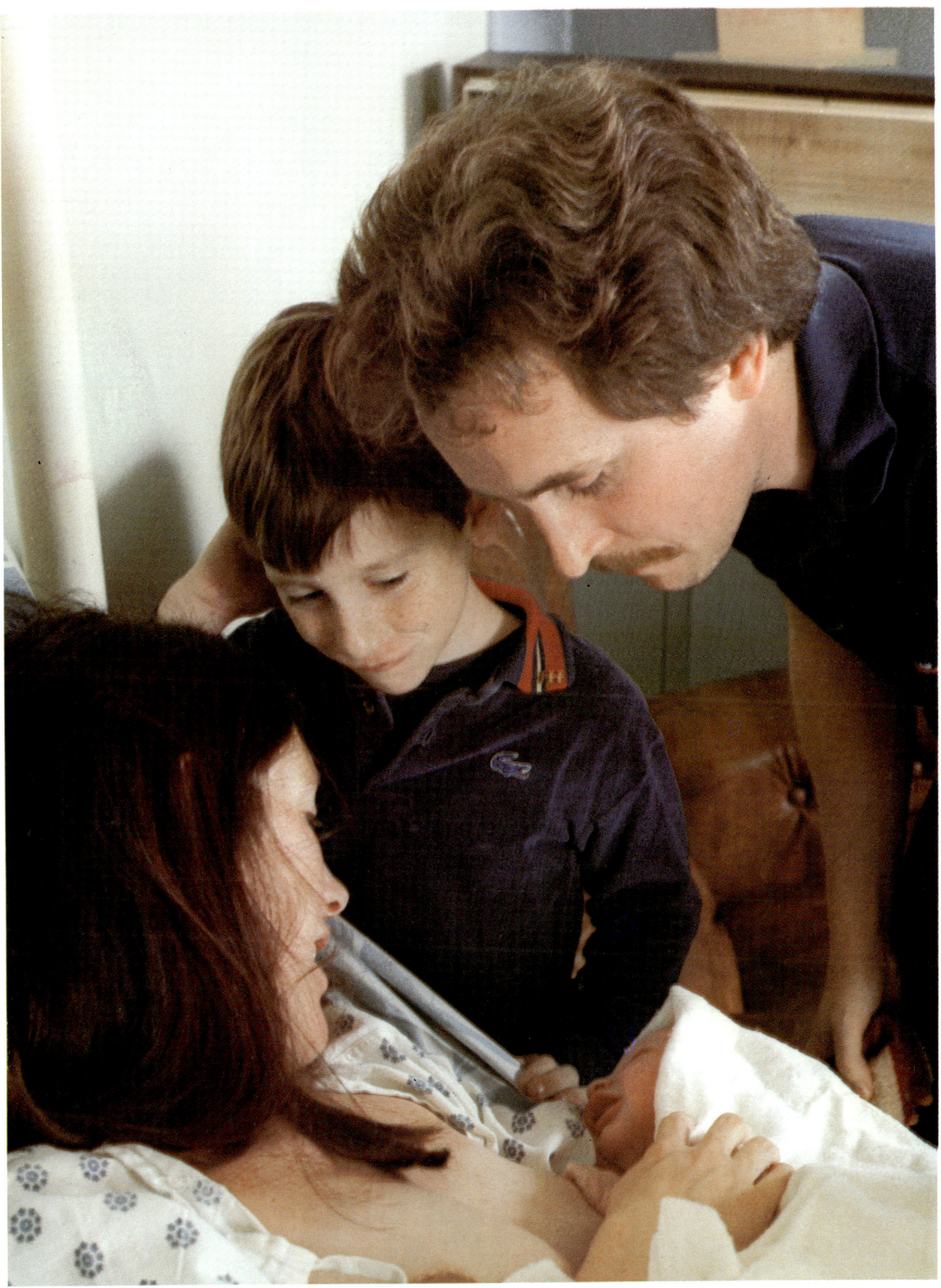

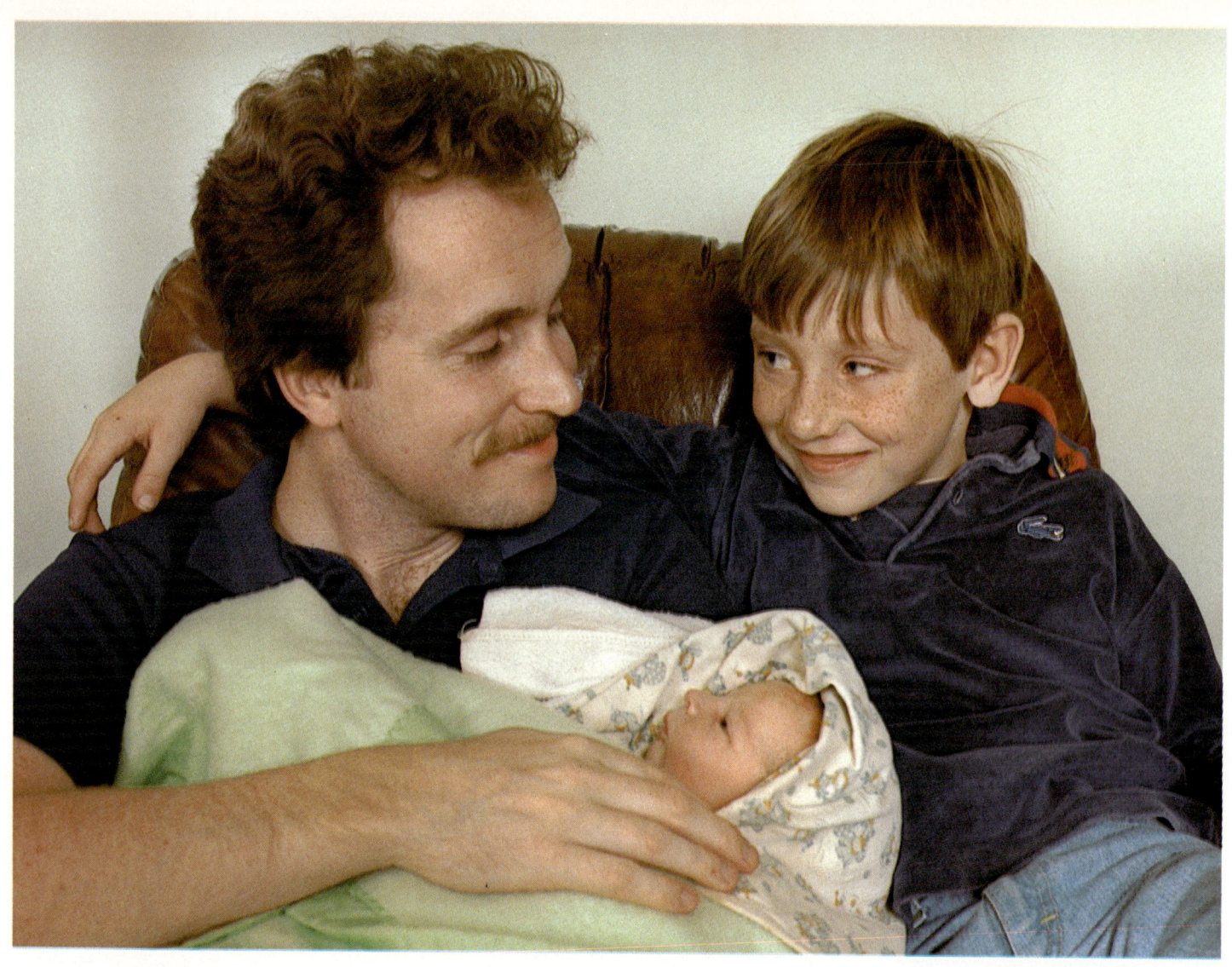

Kenny: Ryan was hoping the baby would be a boy, "so we can get bunk beds." When we told him that he had a baby brother, he went berserk. He was so happy! He wanted to touch him, hold him, and talk to him. He talked to the little guy a lot. Kris responded to Ryan, and seemed to feel comforted by him. Having my two boys together like this was great.

Ryan: As soon as I saw Kris, I loved him right away because I knew he would be my brother forever.

Ellen: How often do people get something this good in life? This is everything I've dreamed of.

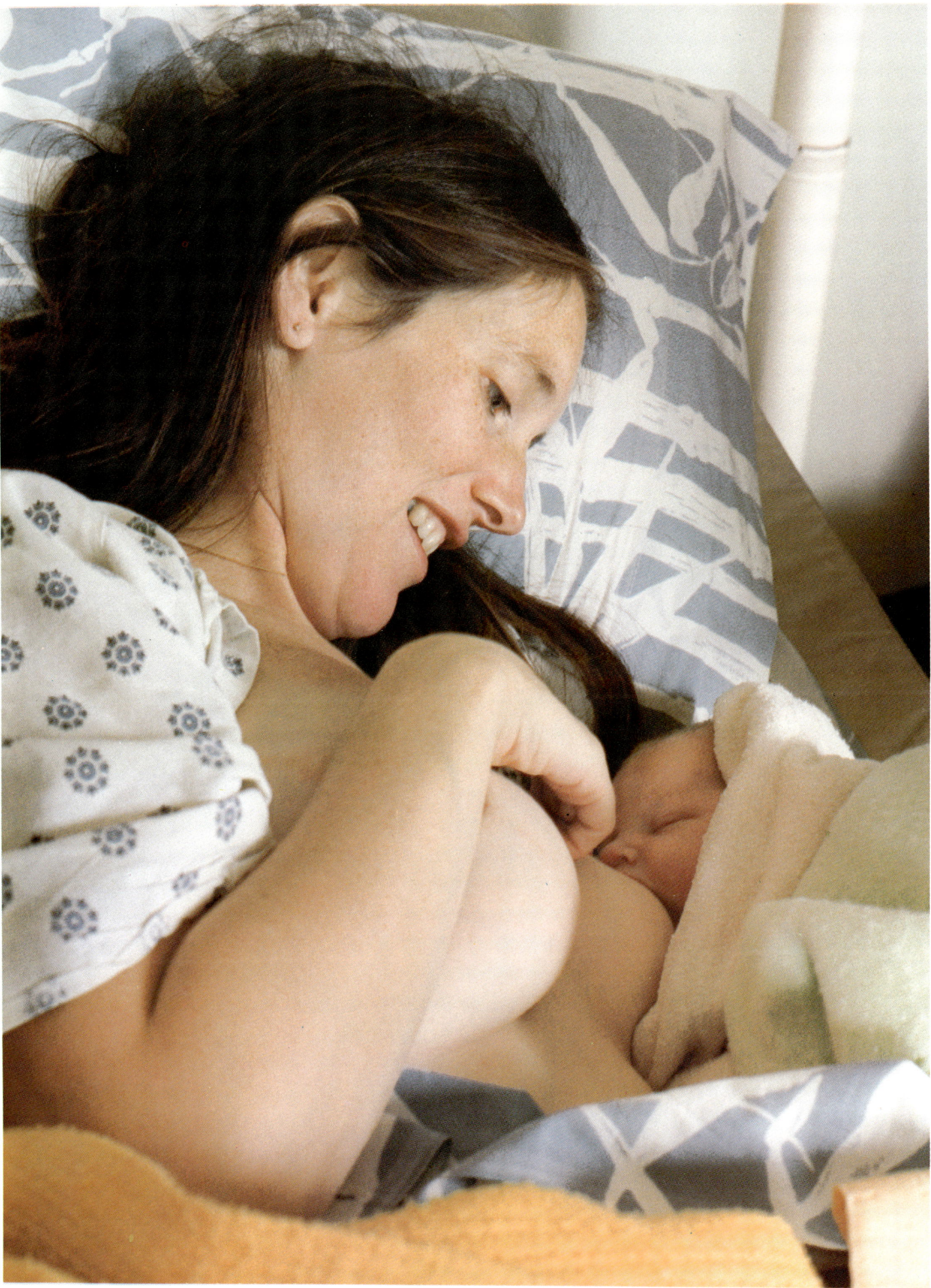

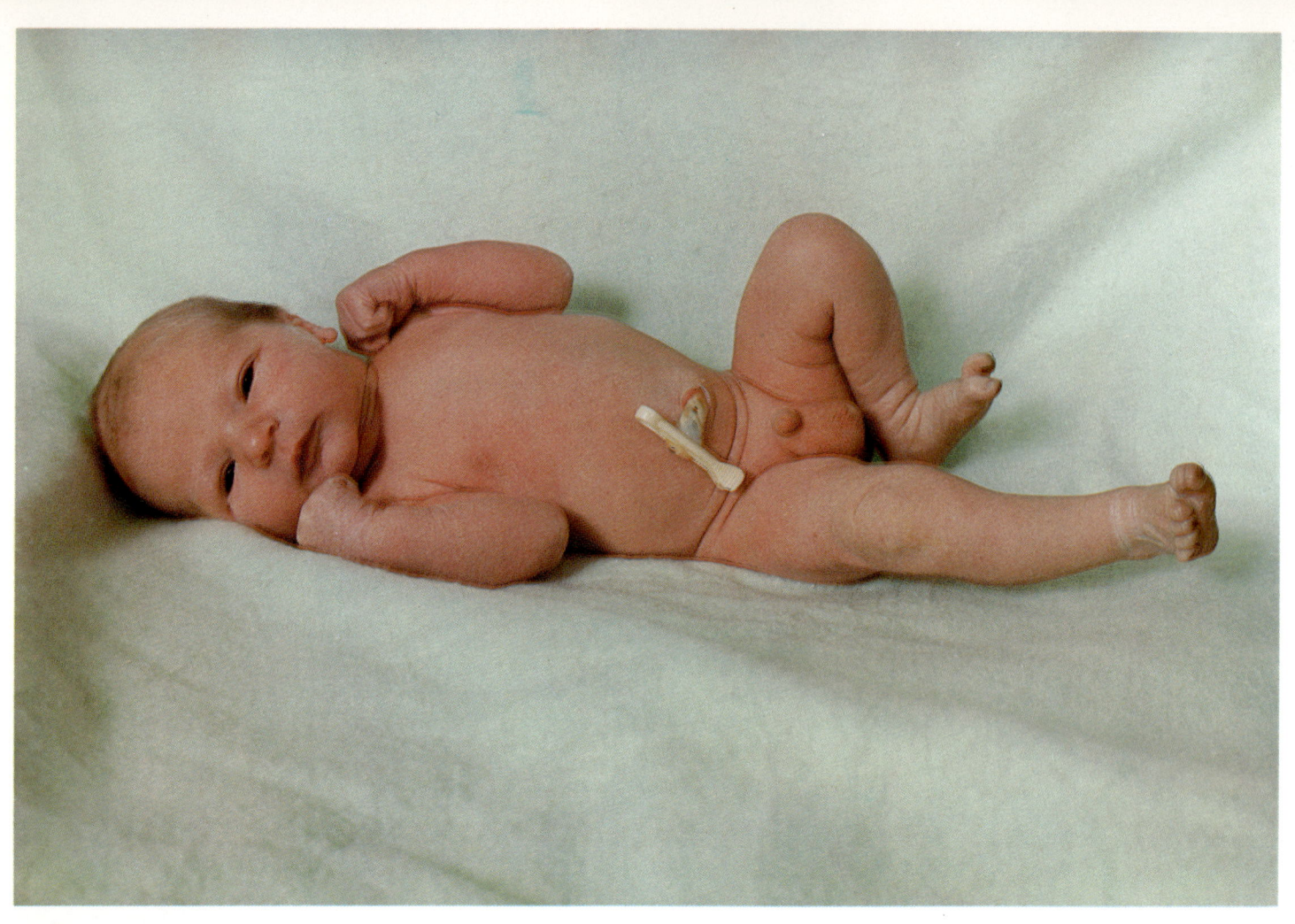

Kris, eight hours old

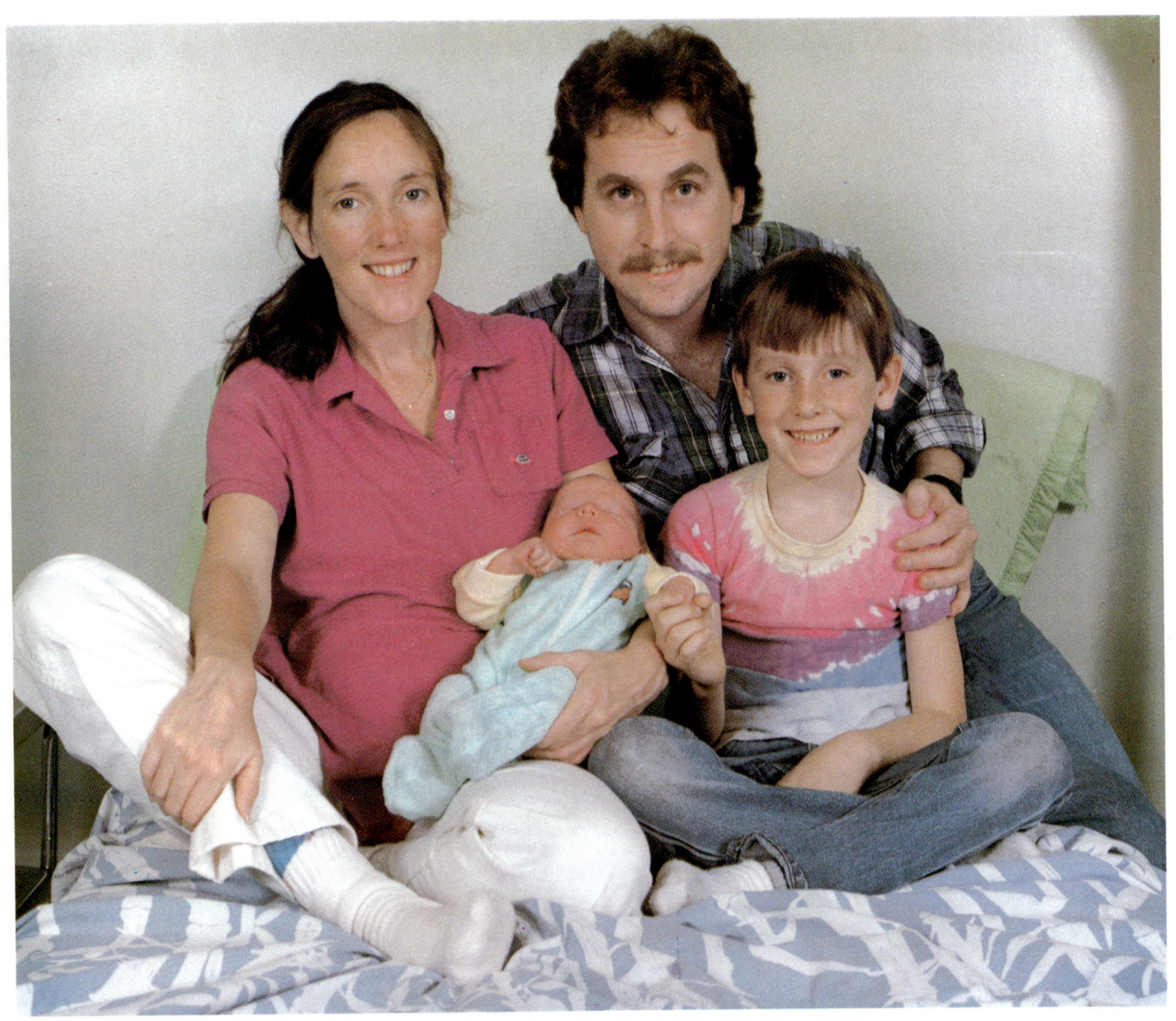

Ellen: Eight hours later, I felt much better. I was still having afterbirth pains, but after some rest and a shower, I was anxious to head on home. We stopped at Kenny's parents' house, and they had a wonderful dinner ready for us. It was so nice to have the family together.

Kenny: A birth like this does so much for the people involved. Sometimes a relationship can wear a little thin during the course of everyday living. But after going through something this emotional together, Ellen and I realized how much we can depend on each other, and we were reminded of all the love there is between us.

PAUL and PAT

Paul: When we first found out that Pat was pregnant, I was excited but I wasn't exactly sure what about. Even when I felt the baby kicking, though I was thrilled, it just wasn't the same for me as it was for Pat, who was actually carrying the baby. The incredible bond that Pat had with this baby could only come from having it growing and developing inside her. At this point, I couldn't possibly feel the same enthusiasm, and that was hard.

Pat: I'd had a really good pregnancy. I was very excited about the baby and couldn't wait for it to be born. But as it got closer to my due date, I began to have some ambivalent feelings about the birth. Every time I felt a contraction, I would hope that I was in labor. But then I thought, "Well, maybe I can hold off for another day."

As a nurse, I'd seen many women go through labor. I knew that while the experience had been very positive for a lot of them, for others it had been terribly painful. I didn't know which category I was going to fit into, and that made me nervous.

Paul: Pat didn't sleep well for two weeks before the birth. Every night, she'd wake me up announcing, "This is it!" Then, because she couldn't sleep, she wanted me to stay up with her.

Pat: He got so fed up that the night it really did happen, he wouldn't wake up!

I'd been very restless the entire evening before I knew I was in labor. Some friends were over watching a movie with us, but I just couldn't sit still. Around two A.M. I woke up with contractions. They weren't regular, but they felt stronger than usual. I started staining around six A.M., and Paul called the Center an hour later.

Paul: Her contractions were unpredictable. She would have two in less than five minutes, then none for almost twelve minutes. I described this to the midwife on the phone. She was very casual, and said to stay home for a while and relax. She said, "With a first baby, especially since the contractions are so irregular, it could be hours before anything much happens."

Pat: My sister-in-law, Linda, and I are very close, so we asked her to be with us for the birth. She's pregnant with her second child, and because she had been through childbirth, I knew that she would be wonderful as an extra support person. She came over around nine A.M., and she and Paul dragged me outside for a walk, saying that it would speed up the labor. It didn't seem to matter to them that it was freezing out, with snow and ice all around. All I wanted to do was go back inside the house when I got hit with a bad contraction. Teasingly, Paul said, "I wonder if this is what they call false labor?" Well, at this point, I was in no mood for jokes. I started yelling at him, "This is not false labor! This is real!"

Paul: An old woman walked by just in time to see me standing with a pregnant lady on either side of me, one of whom was frantic. We went back inside.

At around one P.M., we called the Center again, and I told the midwife that Pat thought it was time to come in. We got there an hour later, and Pat was examined. She was only four centimeters dilated, so the midwife suggested going out to a restaurant, or even a movie, if it was close by. Linda and I were starving, so the three of us went out to lunch.

Pat: I was miserable. Here I was in labor, and it just seemed like everybody was making light of it.

Paul: When we got back to the Center, Pat was examined again, and we found that the labor had progressed significantly. The contractions were coming much closer, but we managed to keep Pat laughing in between them. Within another hour or so, we moved downstairs to the birthing room. I was expecting the room to be very hot for the baby's sake, so I brought light clothing.

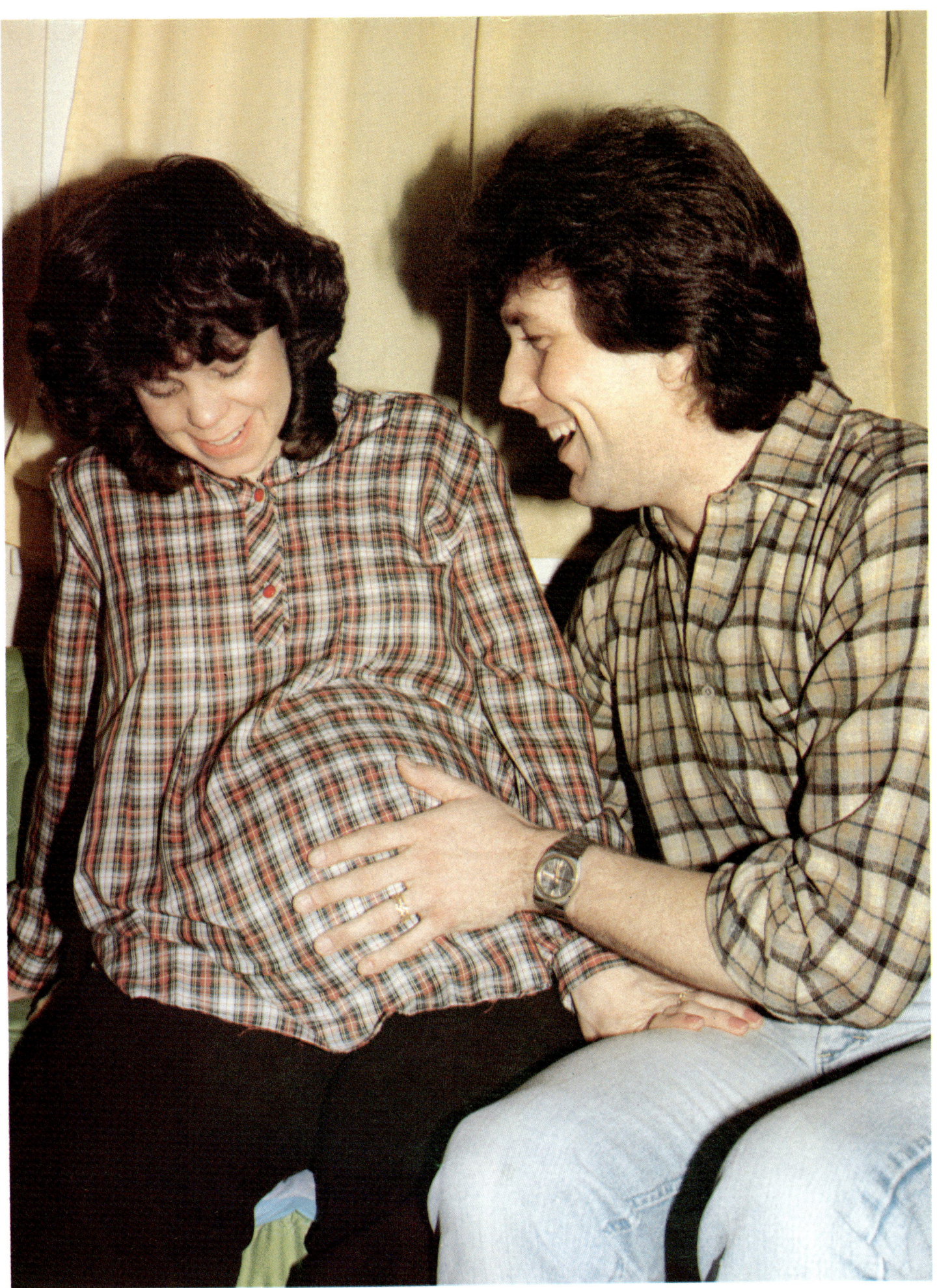

Pat: During the last few months of my pregnancy, I'd thought a lot about the delivery. What worried me most about labor was the idea I might lose control of myself, especially during transition. That bothered me a lot. I've seen some very difficult labors, and the condition that these women get into is frightening. One woman began screaming at her husband, "I hate you for this! Get out!" What if I said something like that to Paul? I would be mortified! I was definitely more concerned about acting crazy than any pain that would make me that way.

Paul: I wasn't a bit worried about her losing control. If she lost her head, I would just help her get her composure back. Besides, I had an enormous amount of confidence in Pat, and I knew that she would be fine.

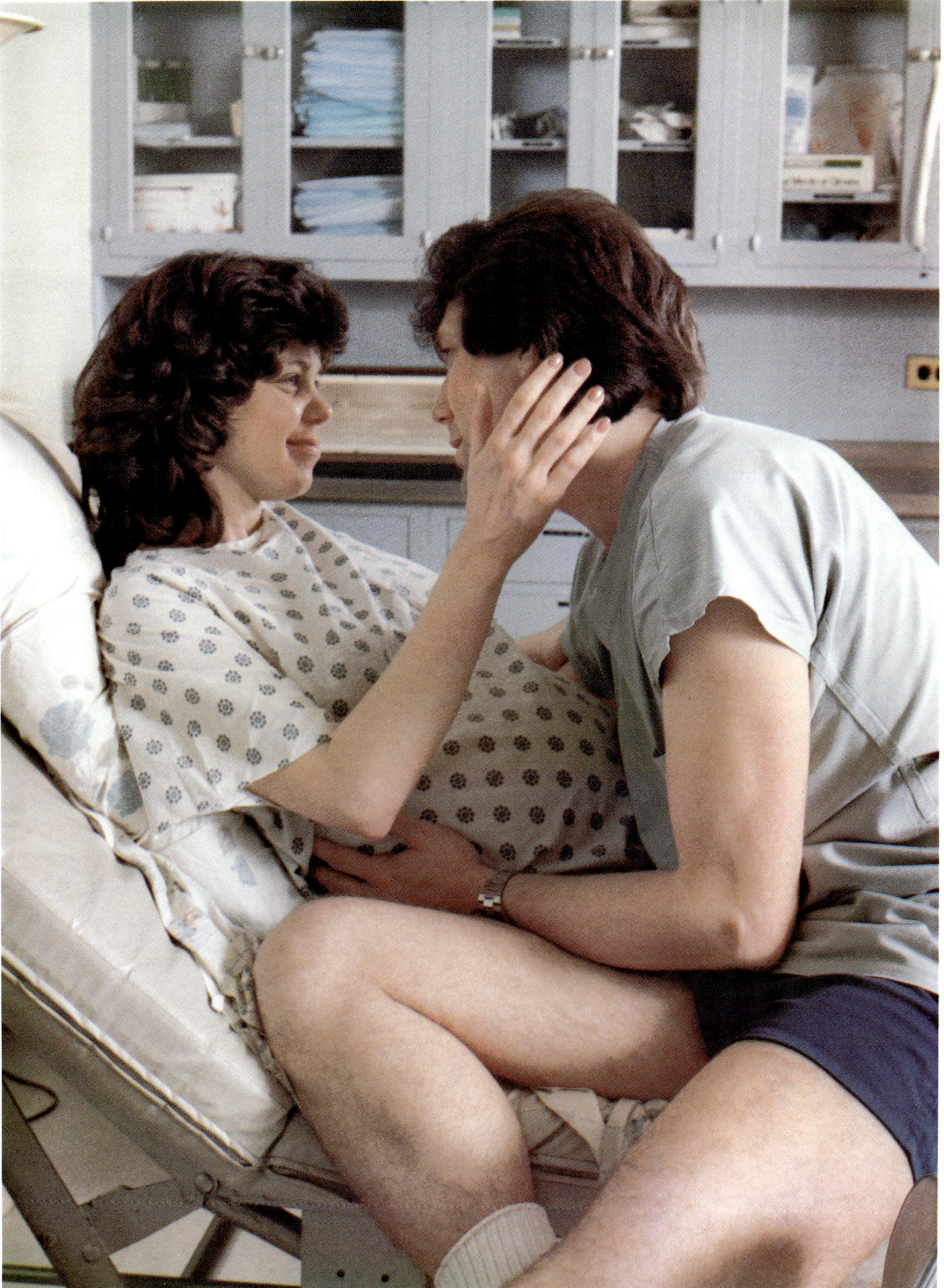

Pat: At this point, I was getting very tense. I didn't know why, but I started crying. There was pain, but that wasn't it. Maybe I was frightened, but in any case, it was only for a brief moment.

Paul: I just felt really terrible for her. I knew that all the comforting in the world could only do so much until the baby was born.

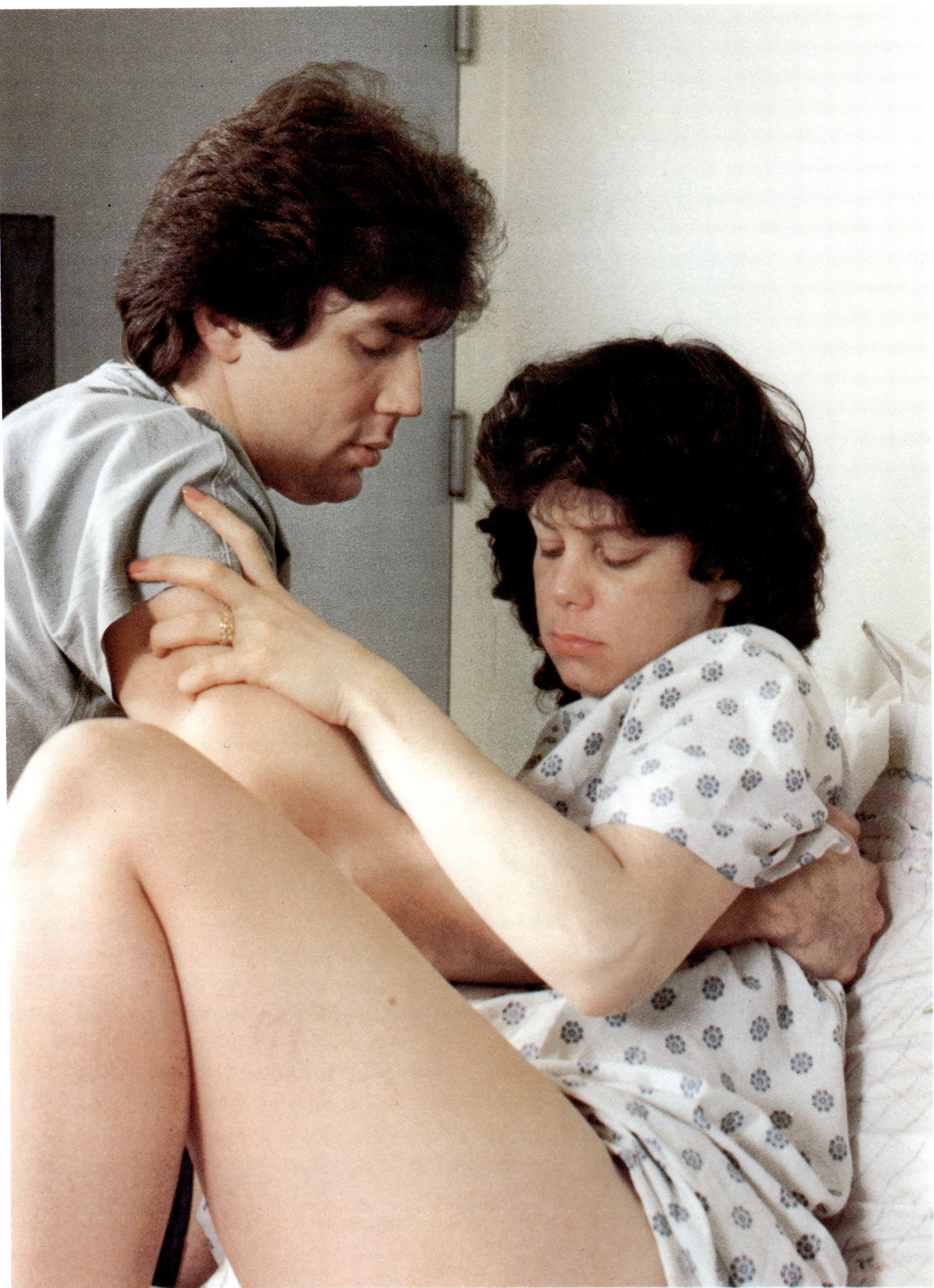

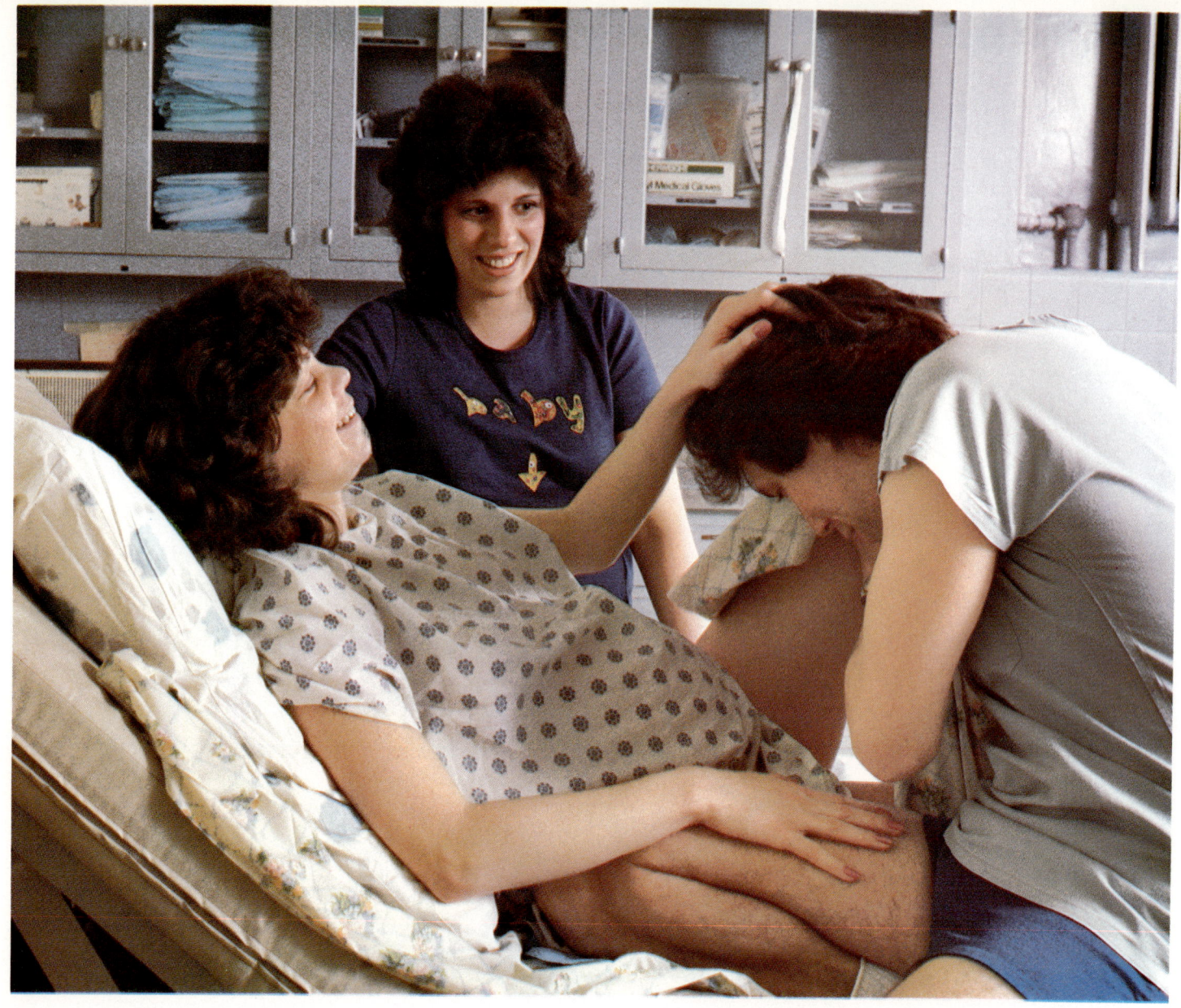

Paul: I tried to make her laugh to break the tension. I guess it's always been my way.

Pat: That was very helpful. He started talking to the baby. He said, "Hello in there. This is your father speaking. We're anxious to meet you. Could you please hurry out?"

I wasn't too concerned about losing control anymore. I was too busy thinking about being uncomfortable, mostly because I kept expecting it to get worse. But it never really did.

Paul: These contractions were very strong, but Pat found a good way to get through them. Each time one started, I would help her to sit up and rock back and forth. She rocked as hard as she could until the contraction subsided.

Pat: The contractions were almost one on top of the other now. Then Linda explained, "It can't get any worse because this is transition." Once she said that, I knew I would be fine.

Paul: I wasn't as nervous as I thought I was going to be. I was determined to keep everything in perspective so that I could remember as much of the event as possible. Pat was handling things so well, and that made it easy to stay calm.

Pat: My water still hadn't broken, and I could feel the baby's head being pushed and meeting resistance with each contraction. I asked the midwife to rupture the membranes. As soon as she did, I felt a tremendous urge to push. But I wasn't fully dilated and was instructed not to push yet. That was awful.

Paul: She said, "I can't help it! I have to push!" I held her tightly and made her look at me. Linda and I both blew very hard right at her, and got her to blow through the contraction. There was only one bad contraction like that, after which the midwife examined Pat again and said that she was fully dilated.

Blowing to avoid pushing
Occasionally a woman will have an urge to push before she is fully dilated. It is important that she know how not to push. She must blow sharply and continuously throughout the urge. The blowing will prevent her from closing her throat and straining downward. She will not be able to stop her uterus from pushing, but she can prevent herself from adding pressure on the uterus.

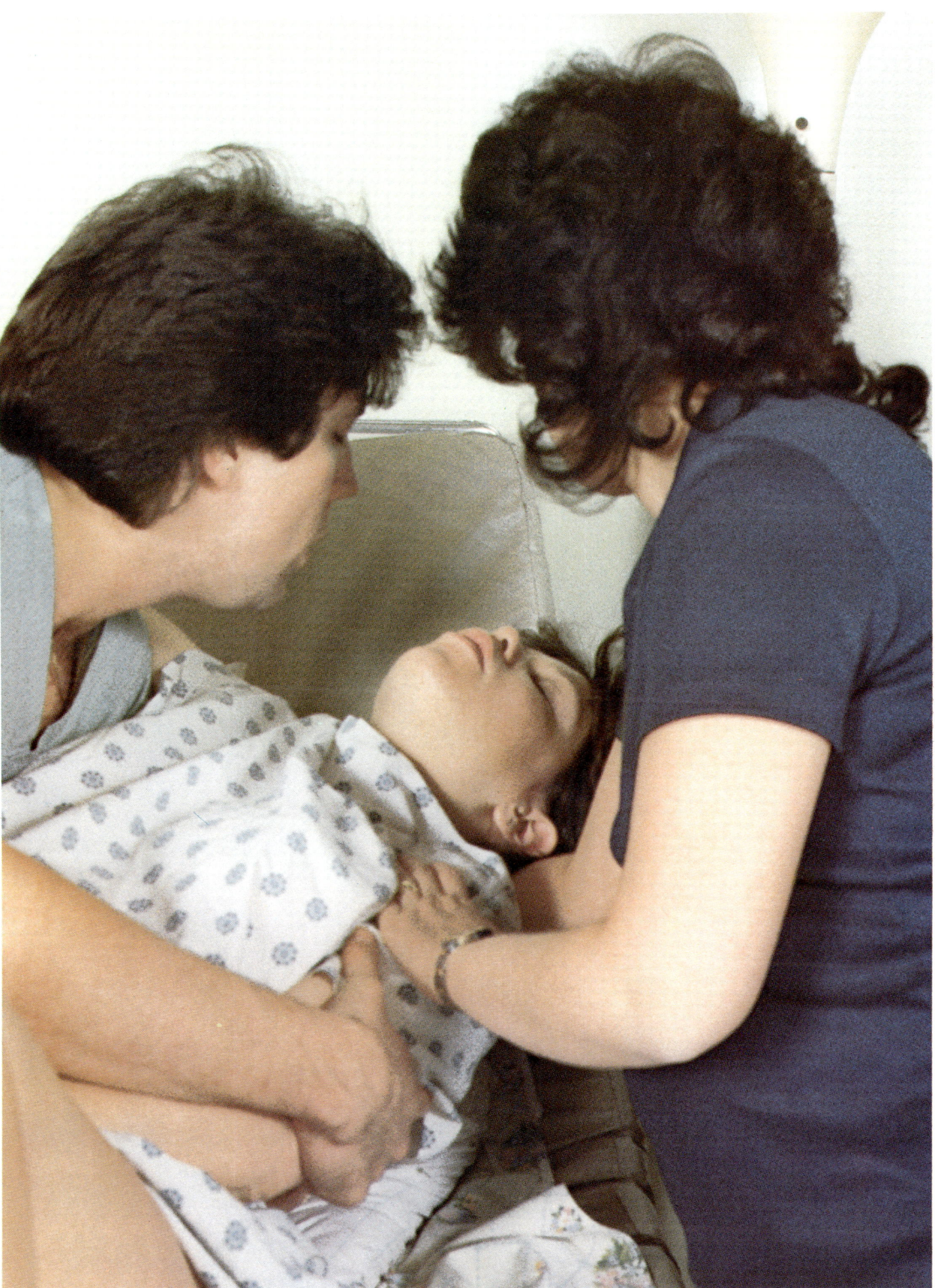

Pat: I remember being asked if I wanted a mirror so I could see the baby come out. At that time, it was the last thing on my mind. As the baby started stretching its way out, it hurt and burned terribly. All I wanted to do was get that baby out and have it be over with.

Paul: The baby was born very quickly. With Pat's first push, the baby's head appeared, but I didn't recognize what it was. For one thing, it was gray, so I didn't think it could be the baby. I don't know whether I expected the baby to come out fully clothed or what. I guess I thought the head would be beige or brown, like hair.

As the head started to crown, I realized that it was the baby, and that this was it! Instantly, the exceptional calm that had remained with me throughout the labor was gone. My head filled with all the fearful thoughts that I tried to avoid. I forgot all about the sex of the baby or the names we had chosen. All I could think about was whether or not the baby would be all right.

But after the baby's head crowned, I got completely caught up in the excitement of the birth.

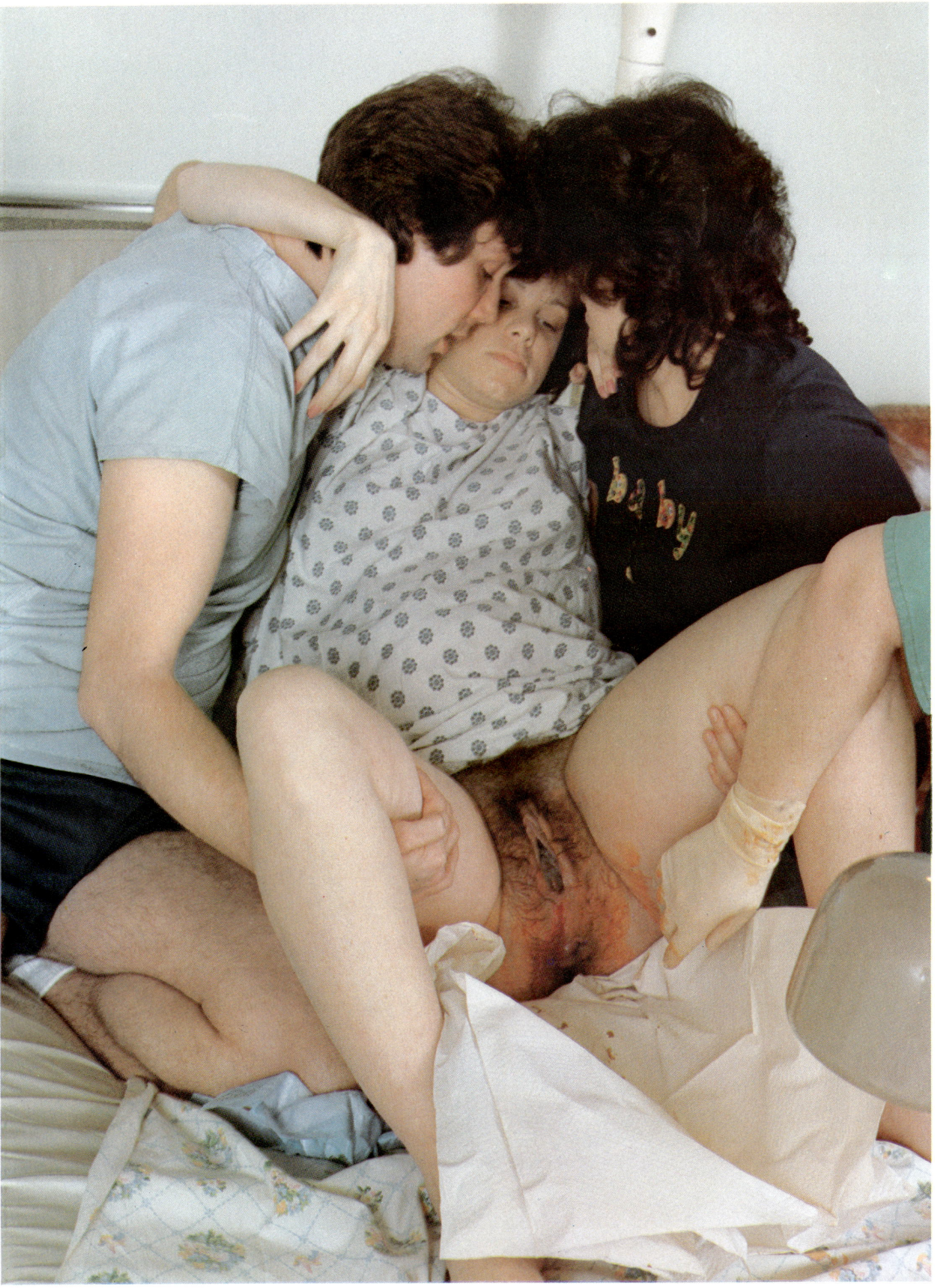

Paul: This part was the most painful for Pat. It was hard to take my eyes off the baby, even for a second, but I wanted to reassure Pat as best I could.

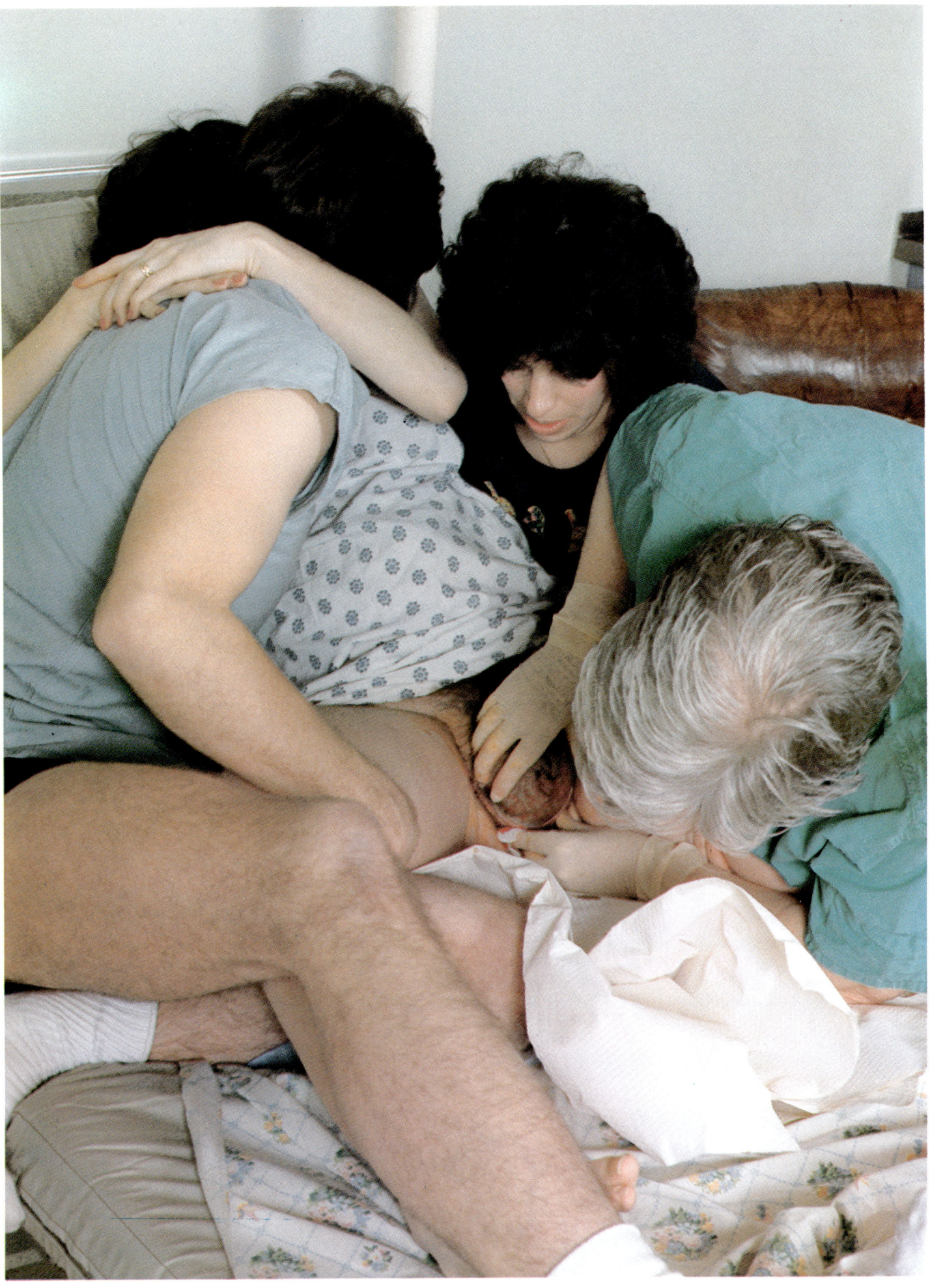

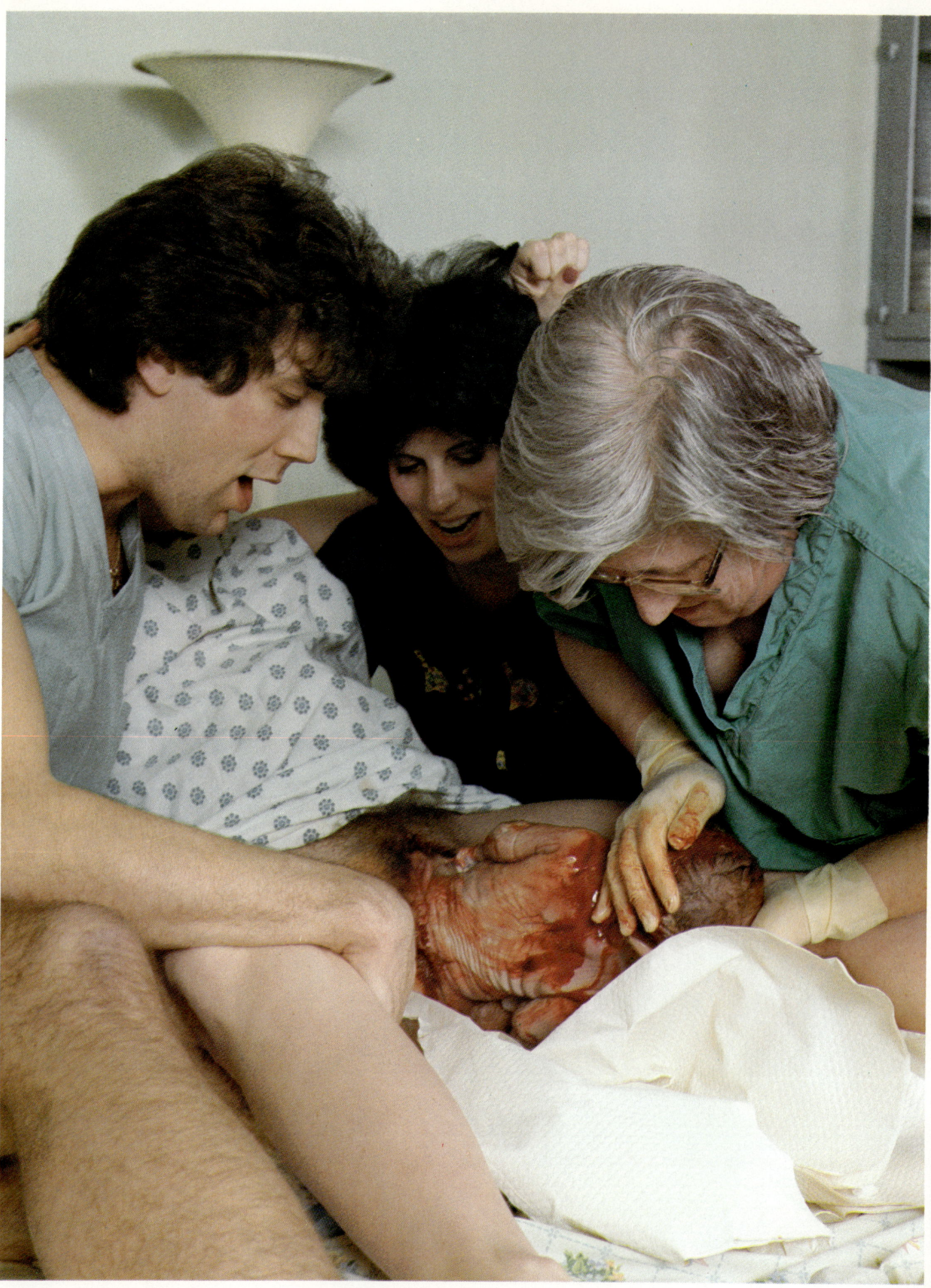

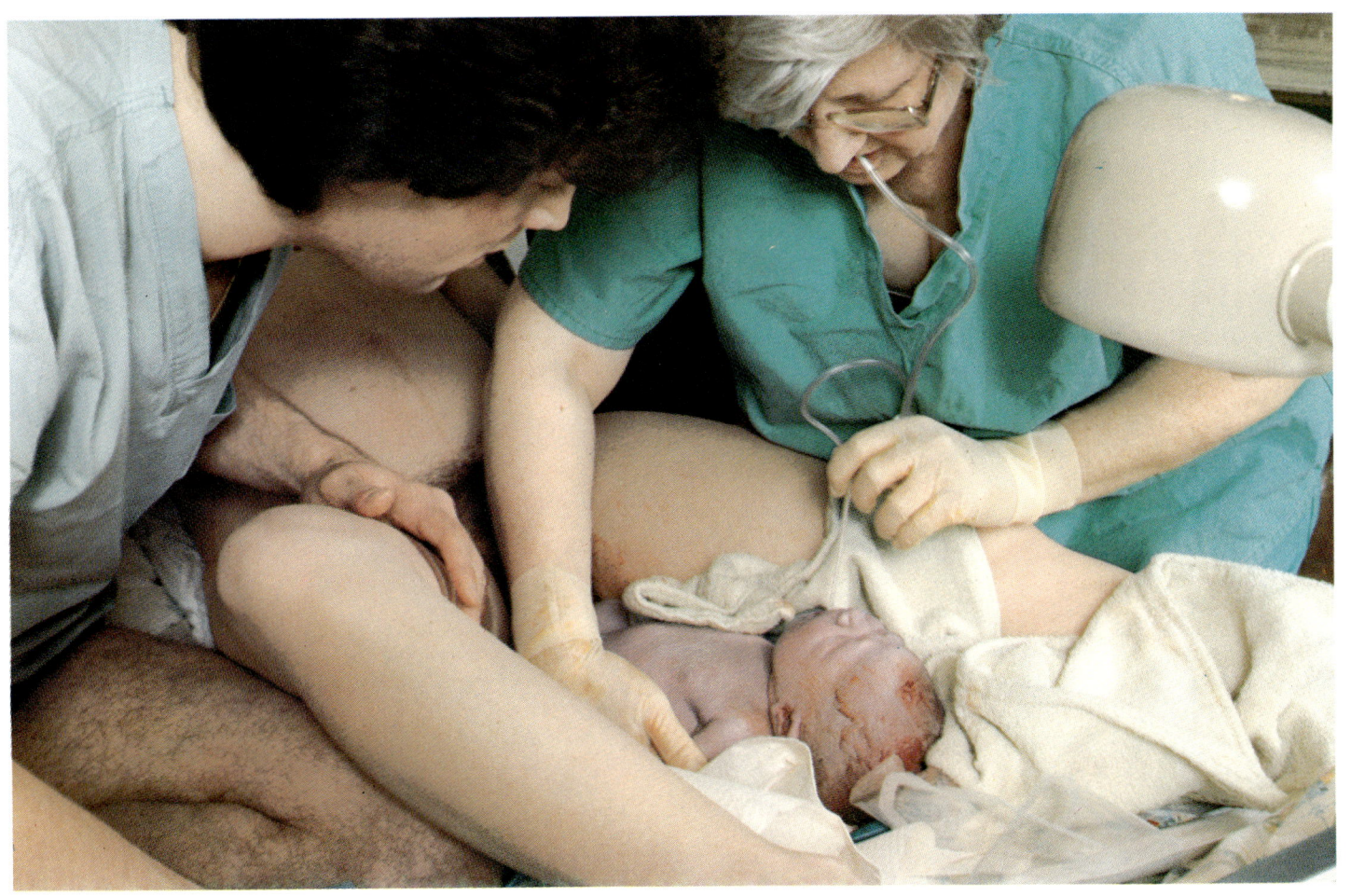

Paul: I was thrilled out of my head! But then I noticed that the baby wasn't breathing. It wasn't moving or anything. It lay very still, and I began to panic.

Realistically, it was only a minute or so before the baby was suctioned out and breathing, but for what seemed like an hour, I was scared to death.

Once I knew that the baby was all right, I looked down and saw it was a girl. I couldn't believe that I had a little girl! This was my daughter! Then slowly she started to cry, and my fears were replaced by more joy than I had ever felt.

Pat: He called out, "It's an Alison!" and I thought, "Now I have my little girl."

The baby's first breath

The moment the baby is born, the doctor or midwife will help it breathe by aspirating the fluid that accumulated in its nose and mouth while it was in utero. The fluid is sucked out with a bulb syringe. Sometimes it may be necessary to use a small rubber tube which can be inserted further into the baby's larynx.

Often the baby will breathe spontaneously. Occasionally the baby will seem quiet and still for a few moments until the fluids are aspirated. This can be frightening for the parents, but it is rarely longer than a minute or two before the baby draws a deep breath.

Paul: I felt such gratefulness to Pat for what she had done. Finally I could fully appreciate what the pregnancy and delivery meant.

Pat: He kept thanking me for the present that he said I gave him.

Paul: I just can't imagine men in this generation not wanting to be there for their own baby's birth. It's such a tremendous loss, and one that they can never recoup. For me, it was definitely the greatest phenomenon I had ever encountered.

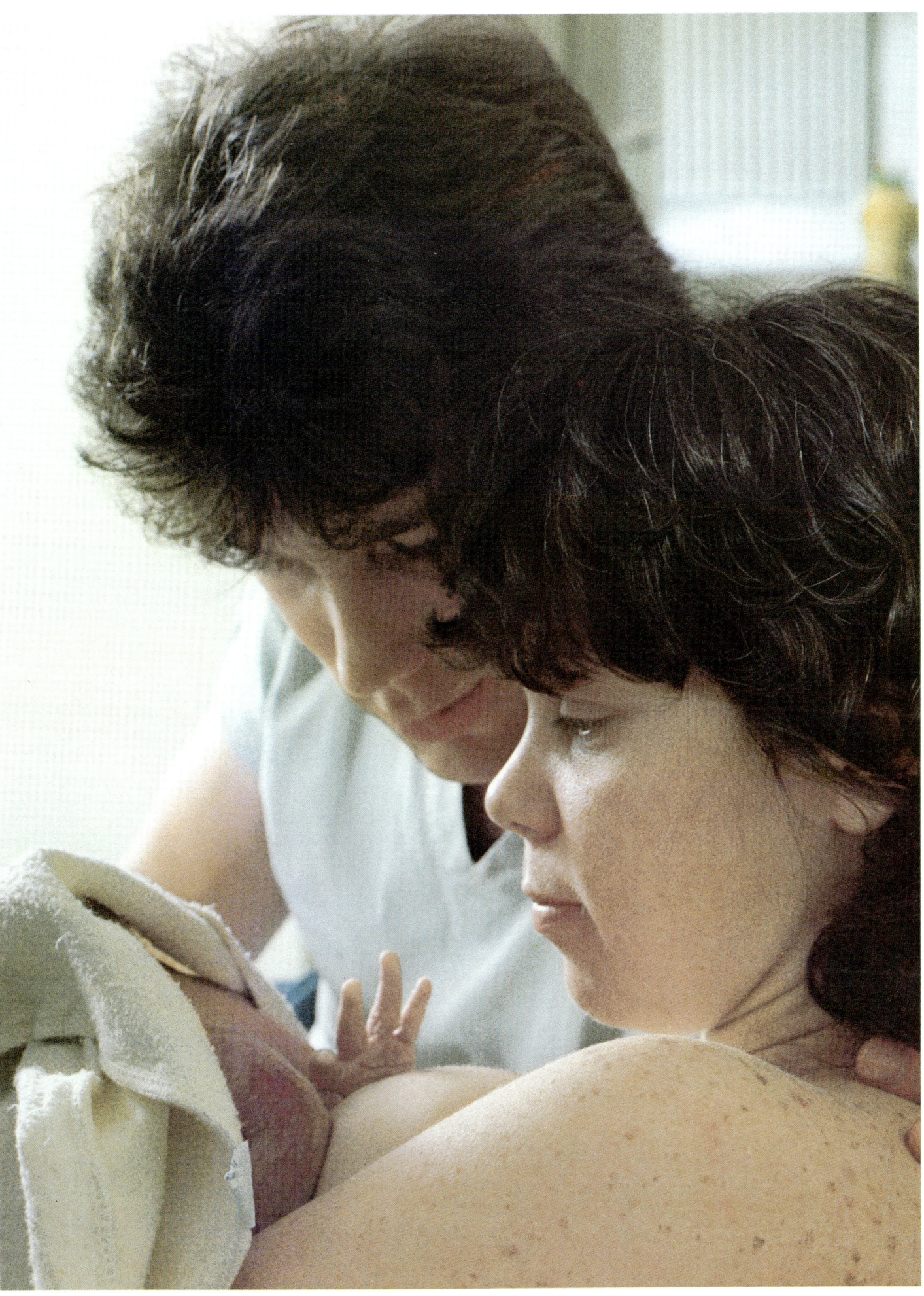

Pat: I was so happy that she was a girl. It meant a lot to me to have a daughter. I was surprised to see how big she was. The doctors kept telling me that the baby felt small, then out came this chubby little thing.

Mostly I was just so excited to finally meet her. I felt like I knew her very well already. While I was pregnant, if I was alone in my office without much to do, I'd play with the baby. I would push on my stomach to see what her reaction would be. She would kick frantically, as if to protest the disturbance. I used to tell Paul that she had a terrible temper, because if I woke her up, she got crazy.

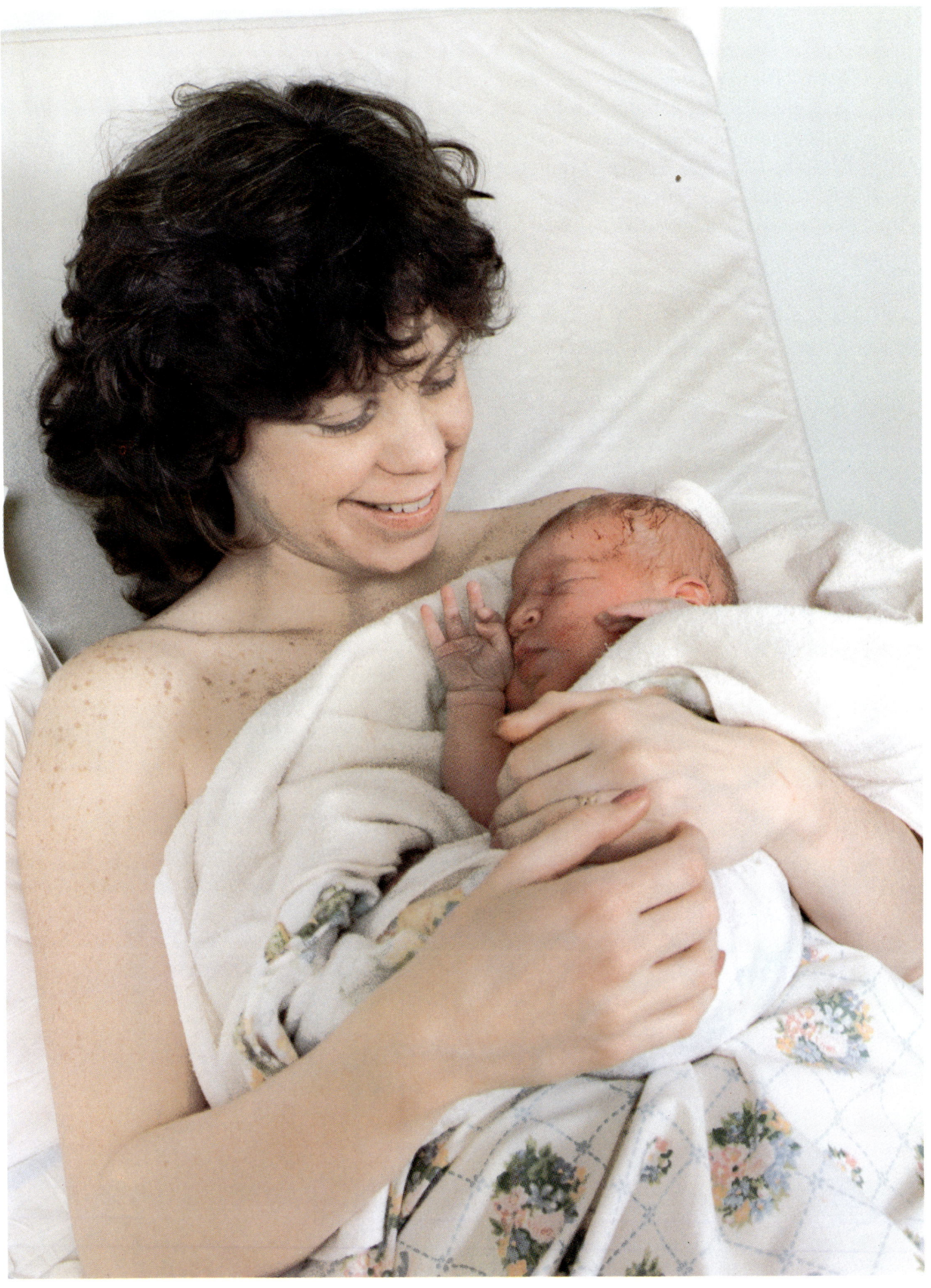

Paul: Now she was really my baby too, and I was going to share in everything that happened to her. As soon as everyone left the room, I unwrapped her and studied her carefully. I couldn't get over how perfect she was! Ten fingers, ten toes; I checked everything out. I held her for hours. I just didn't want to put her down. It was so incredible to believe that this was really my child!

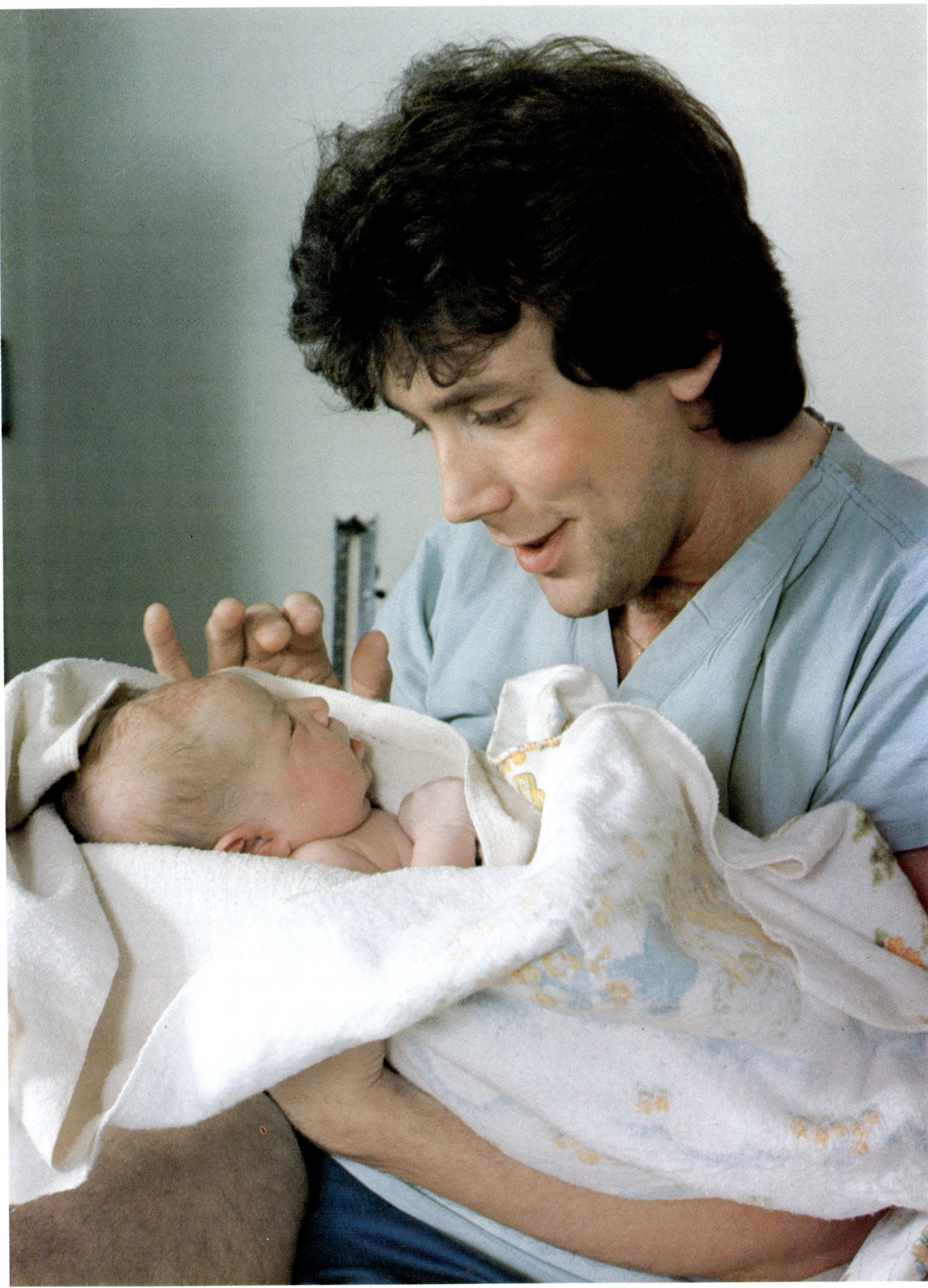

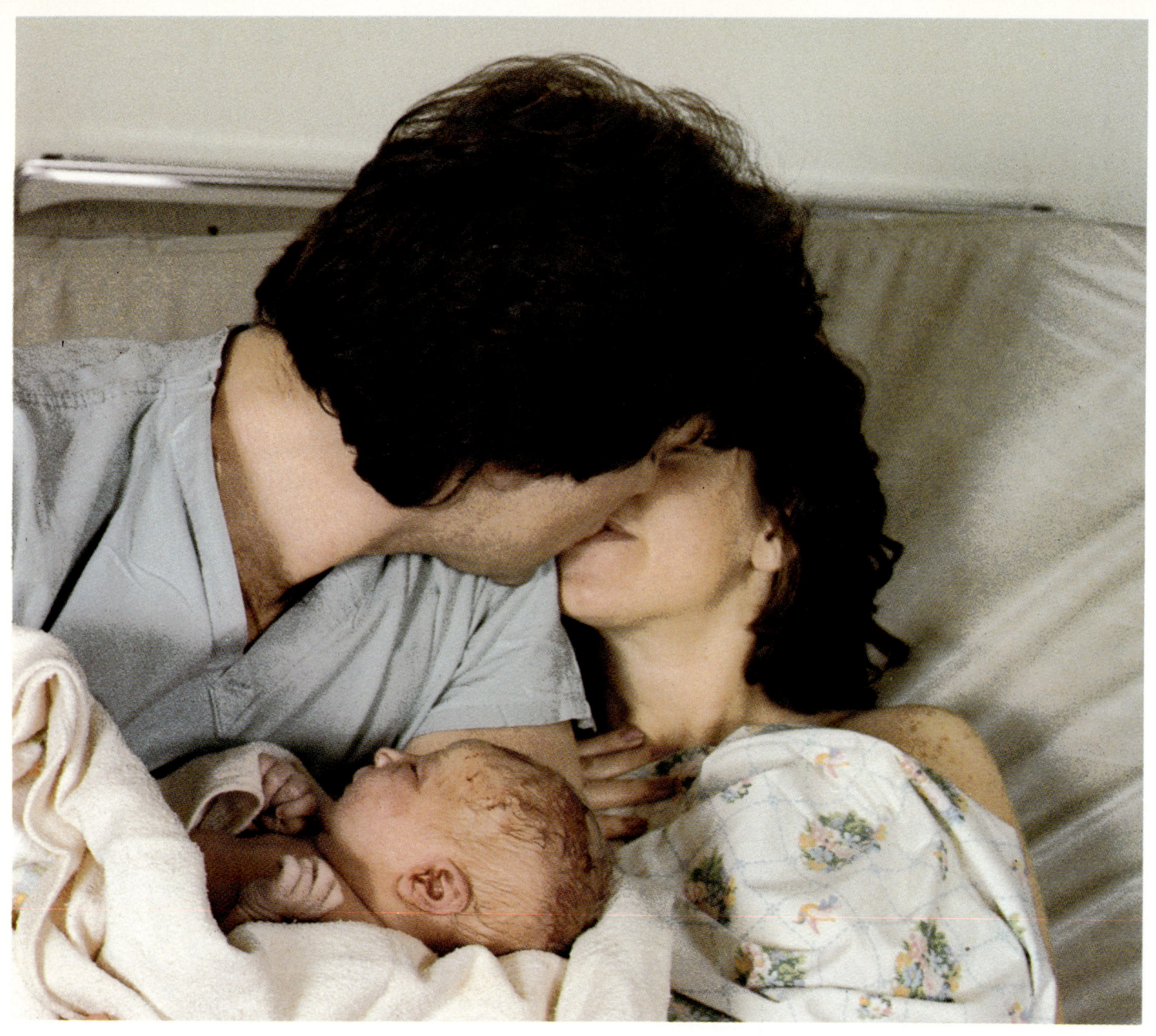

Pat: From the moment Alison was born until we brought her home, she stayed with us. After waiting so long for her to be born, I would have been furious if some nurse took her away. I think it's really sad the way families are so often separated after the birth. The baby goes to the nursery, the father goes home, and the mother is alone. They spend their first night as a family apart from each other, allowing very special moments to be stolen by separation.

Paul: That night I slept in the easy chair, Pat slept in the bed, and our little daughter slept between us in her basket. When she woke up for the first time, I was right there to comfort her, and then Pat nursed her.

SUSAN and DAVID

Susan: This was our first baby, so everything was new to us. We were filled with the wonder and excitement of what was to come, yet there was also some apprehension. Even when things check out, there's always the underlying fear that something might be wrong with the baby. Sometimes it was hard to believe that there really was a baby inside me at all.

David: We got information on the different choices for delivery and found the place that we felt would offer Susan the finest obstetrical care, as well as the safest and most rewarding birth experience. We took childbirth classes together and practiced the breathing techniques.

Susan: At my last checkup with the doctor, he said that the baby had not yet dropped into position, and would therefore probably be late. So even though it was less than a week from my due date, I tried to keep busy with everyday activities.

David and I went to a counseling class, as we often did on Tuesdays. We had paired off separately, and I was working with Andy. It was my turn to listen, and I wanted to give him my utmost attention. This became increasingly difficult to do because I was distracted by a strange leaking sensation that was making my pants slightly wet. I wondered if it meant my water had broken, but it didn't seem like that much. Besides, I couldn't really be having the baby yet. Still, the situation definitely warranted my attention. I hated to interrupt Andy, but finally I said, "I'm sorry, but I must go to the bathroom." As I started up the stairs, I felt a gush of water, which then began running down my pants legs. I went to the bathroom and came out yelling, "Oh my God! David, we're going to have a baby!"

When do the membranes break?
On the average, the membranes break about two thirds of the way through the first stage of labor, which is at around six- to seven-cm dilation. But there is really no telling when they will rupture; they may do so hours before any contractions start, or with the onset of contractions, or at a textbook six- to seven-centimeter dilation. Occasionally, the doctor or midwife has to break the membranes, when they are already bulging and are holding back the birth of the baby.

It is interesting to know that the water is only the amniotic fluid that is between the widest diameter of the baby's head and the cervix, or mouth of the uterus. The membranes may break in a gush or just leak, and the amount of fluid varies from woman to woman, from two to three ounces to almost six ounces. The rest of this fluid is held back by the head and shoulders, even though they are not very tight plugs. The remaining water will come out in a gush like a waterfall when the baby's head and shoulders emerge. This will make the baby's passage easy and slippery.

David: I knew right away that her water must have burst. We went straight home and contacted the midwife. Ann explained that although the membranes had ruptured, the baby might not necessarily be born for quite a while, especially since this was Susan's first baby. She suggested that we remain at home and call her again in an hour.

Susan: By then the contractions were coming every two to three minutes. I didn't recognize them as being as intense as they were because I had expected they'd be worse. We called Ann back, and she said to come in to the Center.

We got there around one A.M., and Ann examined me. Her feeling was that the baby would not be born for many hours, so we prepared ourselves for the long wait.

I was on the move the whole time. The contractions were unbearable unless I was walking around and doing the breathing techniques. Ann thought I might wear myself out, so she wanted me to lie down and rest for a while. I tried that, but as soon as the next contraction came on, I jumped right up.

The three of us were in the family room, talking and watching TV. For some reason, I couldn't stand to be with anyone during a contraction. I'd leave the room, get through it as best I could, and return when it was over. I wound up going around in circles, visiting with them briefly, then walking around the corridor for each contraction. Ann asked me if I wanted some support, either from David or herself, but seemed to understand why I preferred to be alone.

David: This was frustrating for me. I had planned to be so helpful, but now there didn't seem to be anything I could do for Susan. I tried gently rubbing her back and shoulders, but she just didn't want to be touched then.

Susan: Ann had been examining me every forty-five minutes or so, and the labor seemed to be progressing very slowly. This time, the exam revealed a marked change, so much so that Ann said it was time to move into the birthing room. I was surprised by this because by this time I thought the labor was going to last forever.

The dark line across the abdomen
Susan is in the middle of a strong contraction. You can tell by how stretched and protruding her abdomen has become. When you look closely, you will see a faint line reaching from her belly button up to her chest. This is the seam that connects the oblique and transverse abdominal muscles. In a nonpregnant woman it is called the linea alba, *or white line. Due to the stretching of the tissues during pregnancy, pigmentation occurs, and frequently becomes visible as a dark line across the abdomen. It is then called the* linea negra, *or dark line. It will fade after the baby is born and eventually will not be visible.*

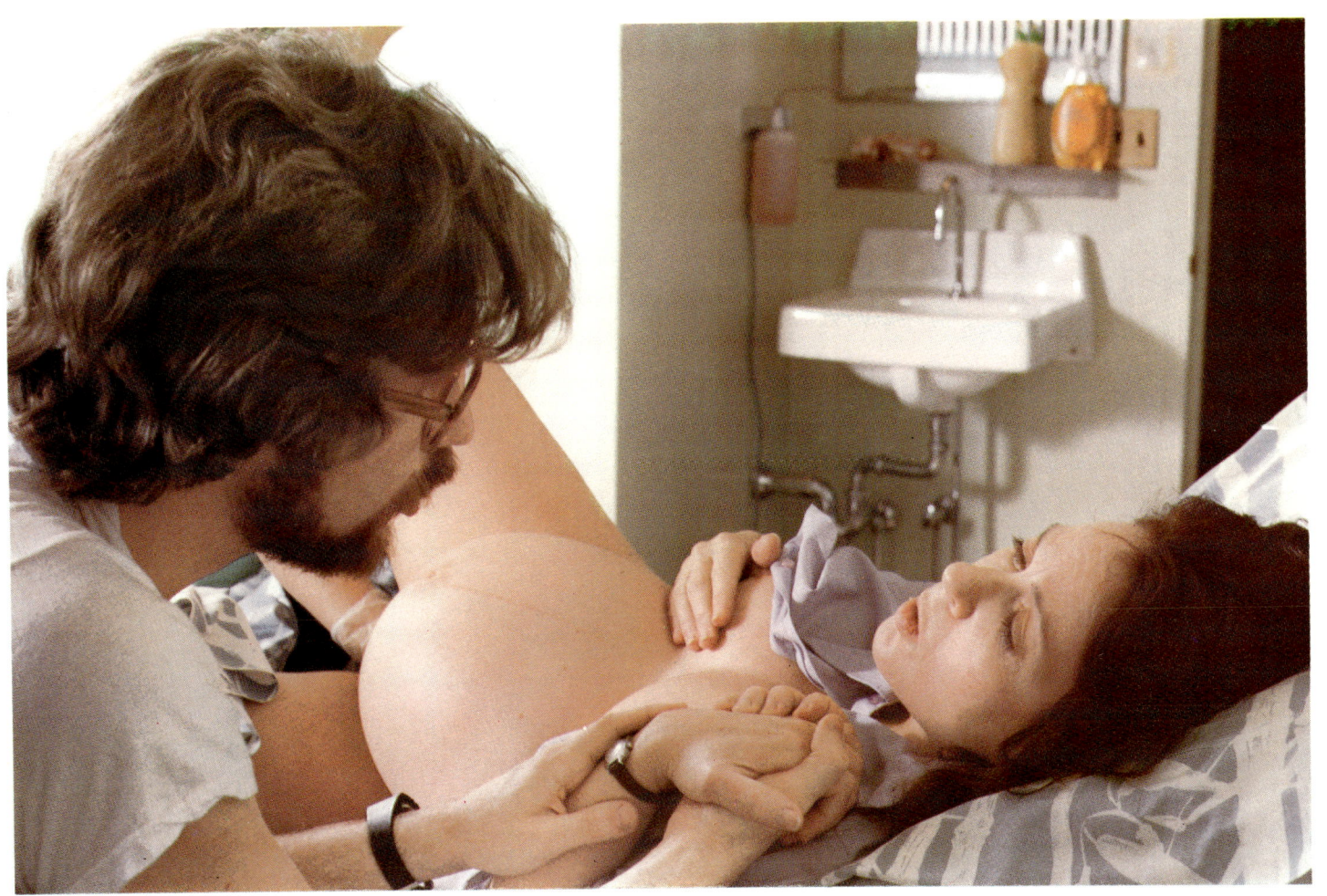

Susan: I was in transition now, and these contractions were very painful for me. I wasn't supposed to push yet, but sometimes it seemed almost impossible not to. David tried to get me through the contractions without pushing. He reminded me to blow and did the breathing with me. He kept saying, "Look at me, look at me!" He was just so intense. Though I was grateful he was doing that, I began to worry he was going to hyperventilate.

David: It's difficult to be so close to someone who's in that much pain.

Susan: I remember feeling he was worried about me, and that was nice. Most of this time was spent just waiting for the next contraction and wondering if I could get through it. Sometimes the breathing really worked, and we could get through the contraction without my losing control. Then I felt sort of elated that I could do it.

David: That was kind of fun and seemed like a real accomplishment.

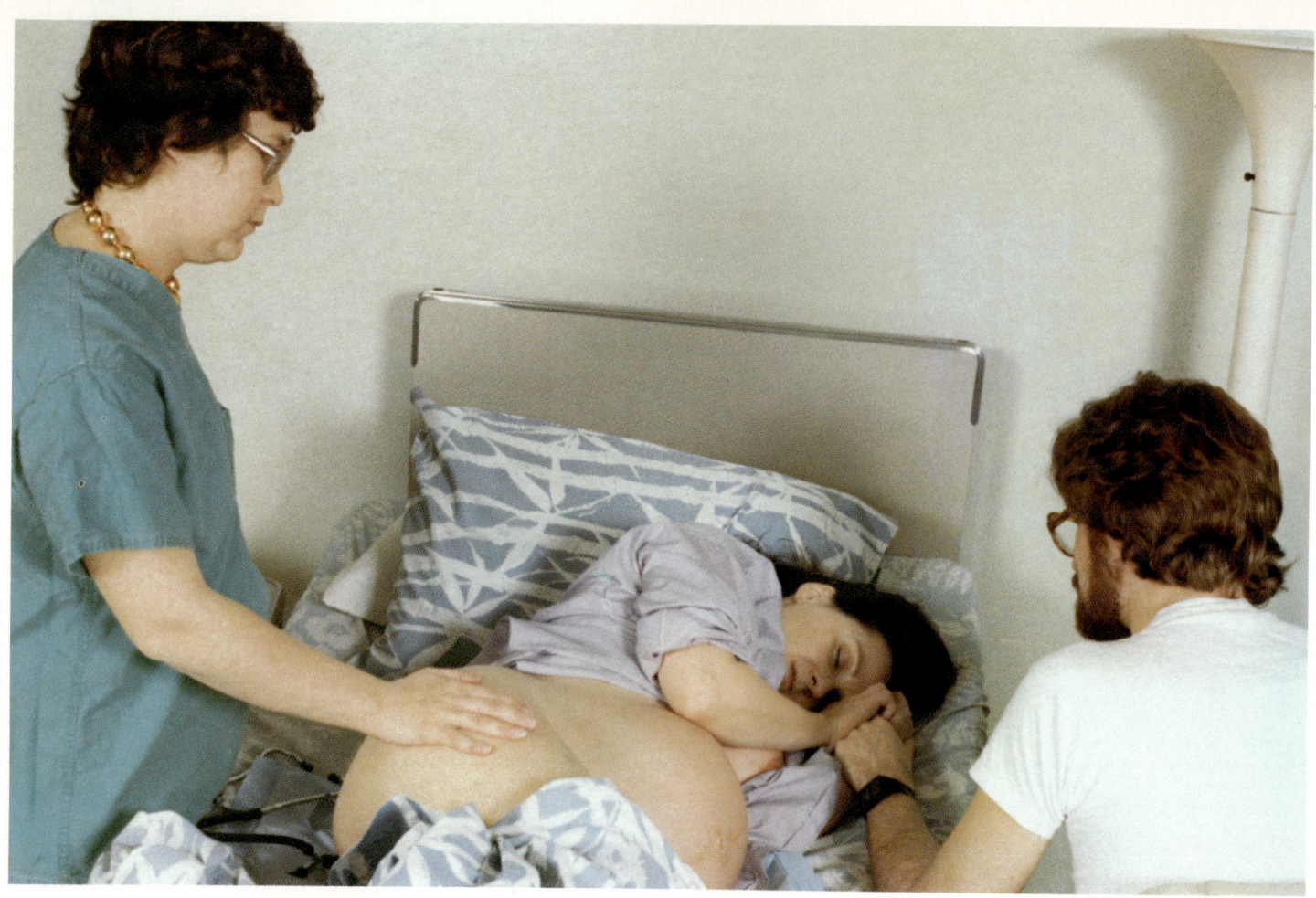

Susan: Just before transition ended, when I wasn't trying to survive a contraction, I remember thinking, "I don't know why I ever did this. If I could undo this pregnancy right now, I certainly would." But then I thought, "There's no way out. I have to go through this."

Ann: Susan, this part of labor is often the most difficult. Transition makes most women feel desperate, and I understand what you're going through. But you're doing fine. Try to remember that it won't be long before you'll be holding your baby in your arms.

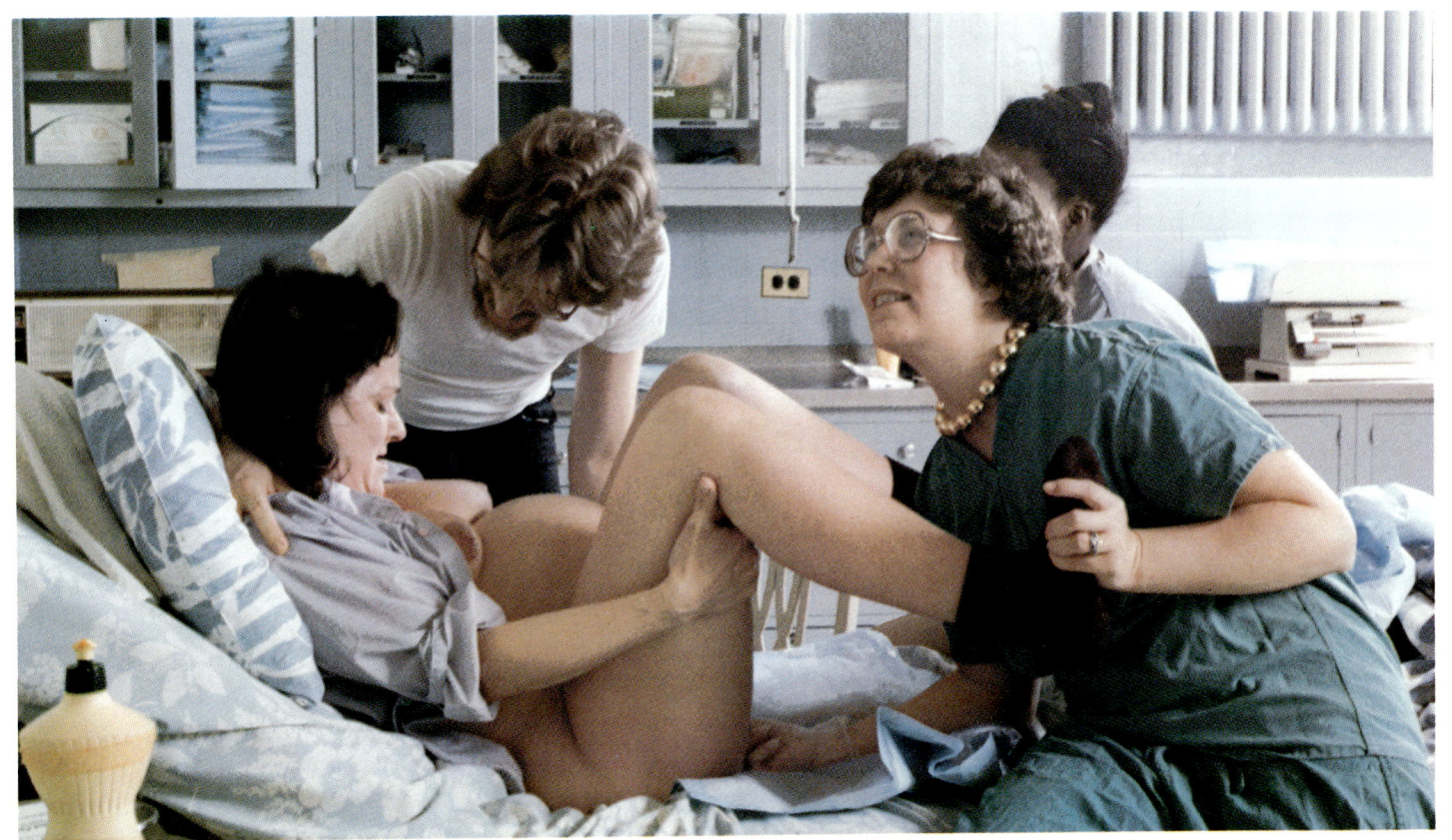

Susan: Finally, at about four A.M., it was time to start pushing. I pushed for quite a while, but nothing much happened. Ann said she could feel that a little bit of the cervix was still covering the head. During the next contraction, she was going to try to slip the rest of the cervix over the widest part of the baby's head. She was able to do this, and the baby came down with my next contractions.

David: Now every time she pushed, we could see the baby's head, but when the contraction was over, the baby would slip back up and out of sight.

Susan: After a while, my uterus began to tire, and the contractions got weaker. Ann said that it was important to make the most out of the contractions, and to try to get three good pushes out of each one. I did this, but the problem was still there. The baby would come down, but instead of coming out, it would slip back up.

David: The level of fear is extraordinary, especially for a couple having their first child. The longer it took, the more worried I became.

Susan: Ann had been checking the fetal heartbeat after each contraction and assured us that the baby was fine. She felt that I could deliver without medical intervention. She also called down another midwife for some new suggestions.

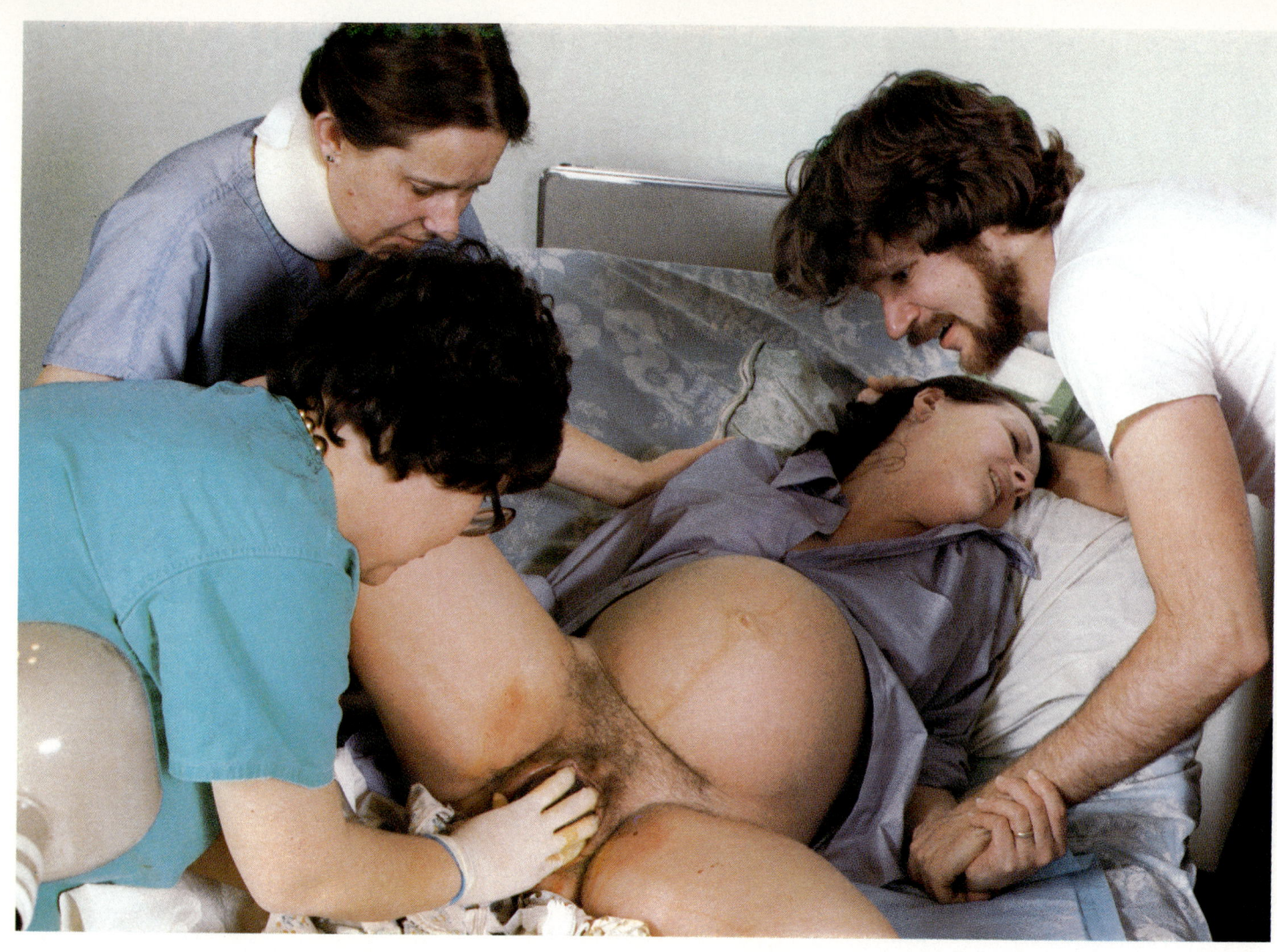

David: Angela [the other midwife] came down and listened to our dilemma. She suggested that with my help, Susan should try a squatting position. I sat in a chair, while Susan squatted on the floor in front of me. I supported her weight from underneath her shoulders. This position was using gravity, so it really made sense to me. Besides, I was very happy that I could work so hard at the labor.

Susan: With David's arms around me, I felt like I could borrow some of his energy. All of a sudden, it seemed as if it wasn't just me pushing the baby out, but both of us together. He was whispering something in my ear like "Come on, darling, push, push!" I could hear in his voice this feeling of "You've got to do it. We've got to get this baby out!" The desperation in his voice kept urging me on. Because he was holding me like that, I was able to push harder than ever, and it worked!

David: That was the turning point. Just before the baby's head crowned, Susan got back on the bed. Then it was only a few more minutes before the baby was born.

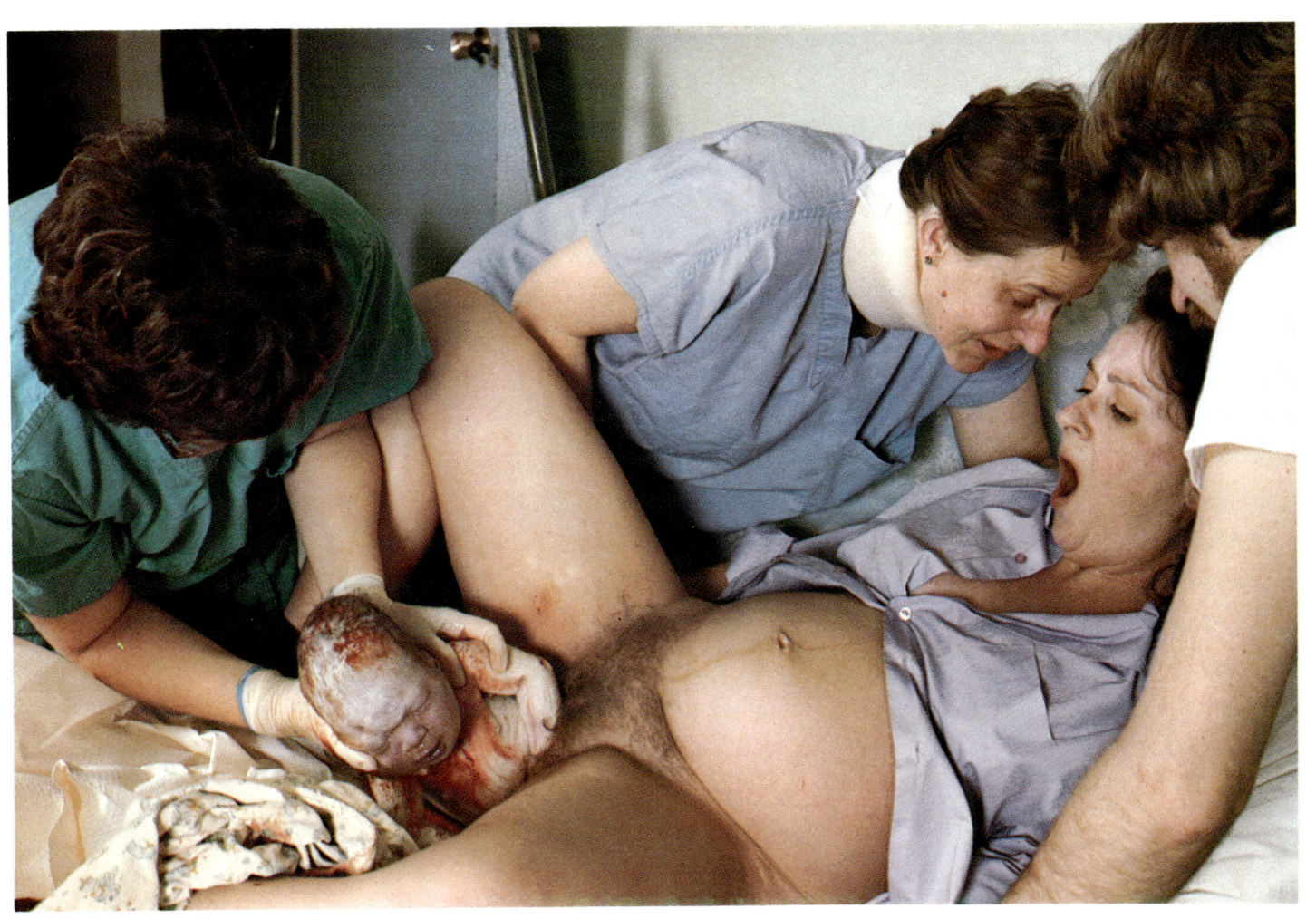

Susan: It was neat having the two midwives there because while Ann was delivering the baby, Angela was giving me a running commentary. She leaned over and said, "Your baby's coming out!" I sat up quickly just in time to see my baby as it was coming out of my body!

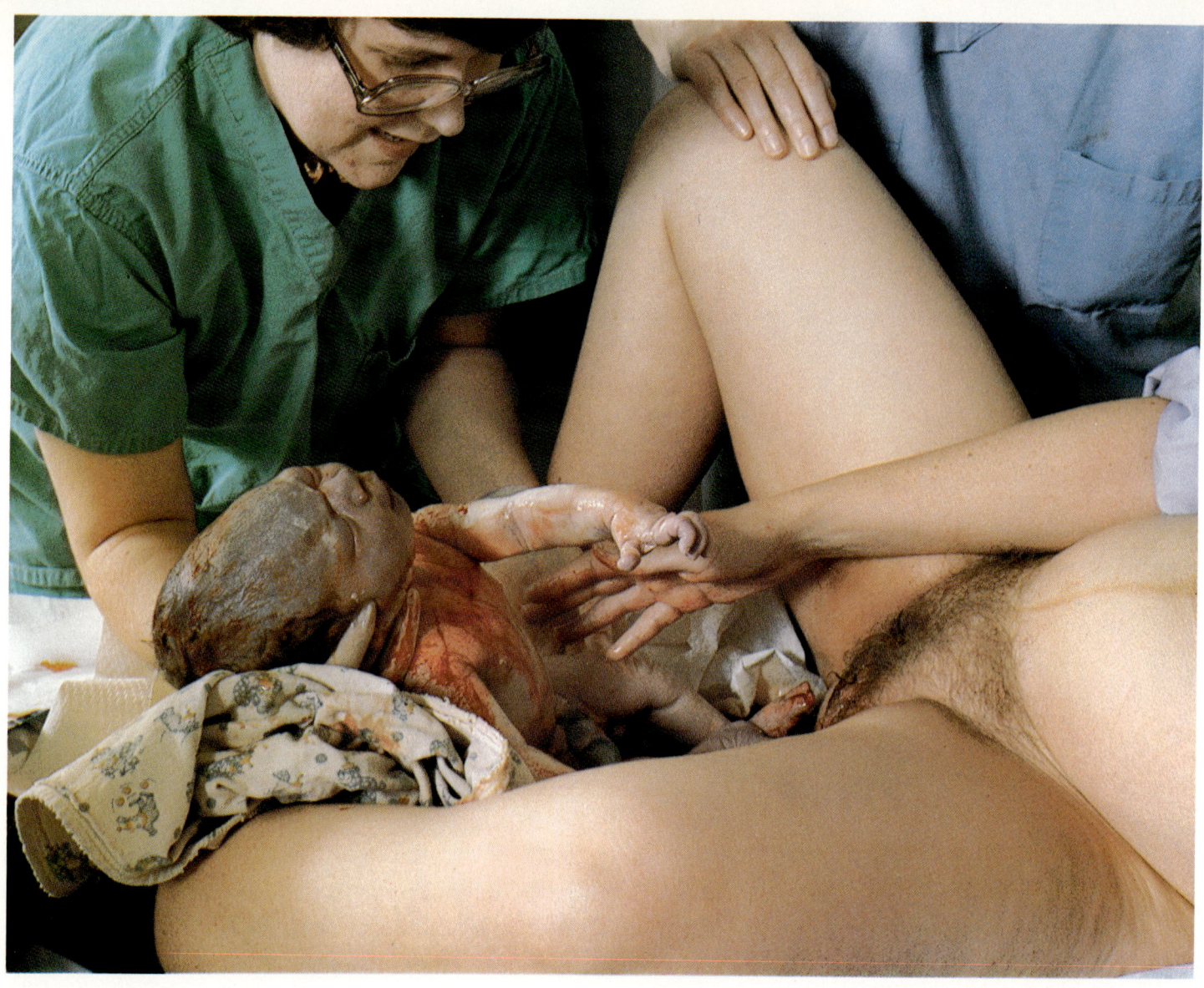

Susan: I felt this little hand. And that's when I first saw its face. I couldn't believe there was actually this little person inside me until I finally saw the face. The whole thing was just so miraculous to me.

I remember David said, "We did it!"

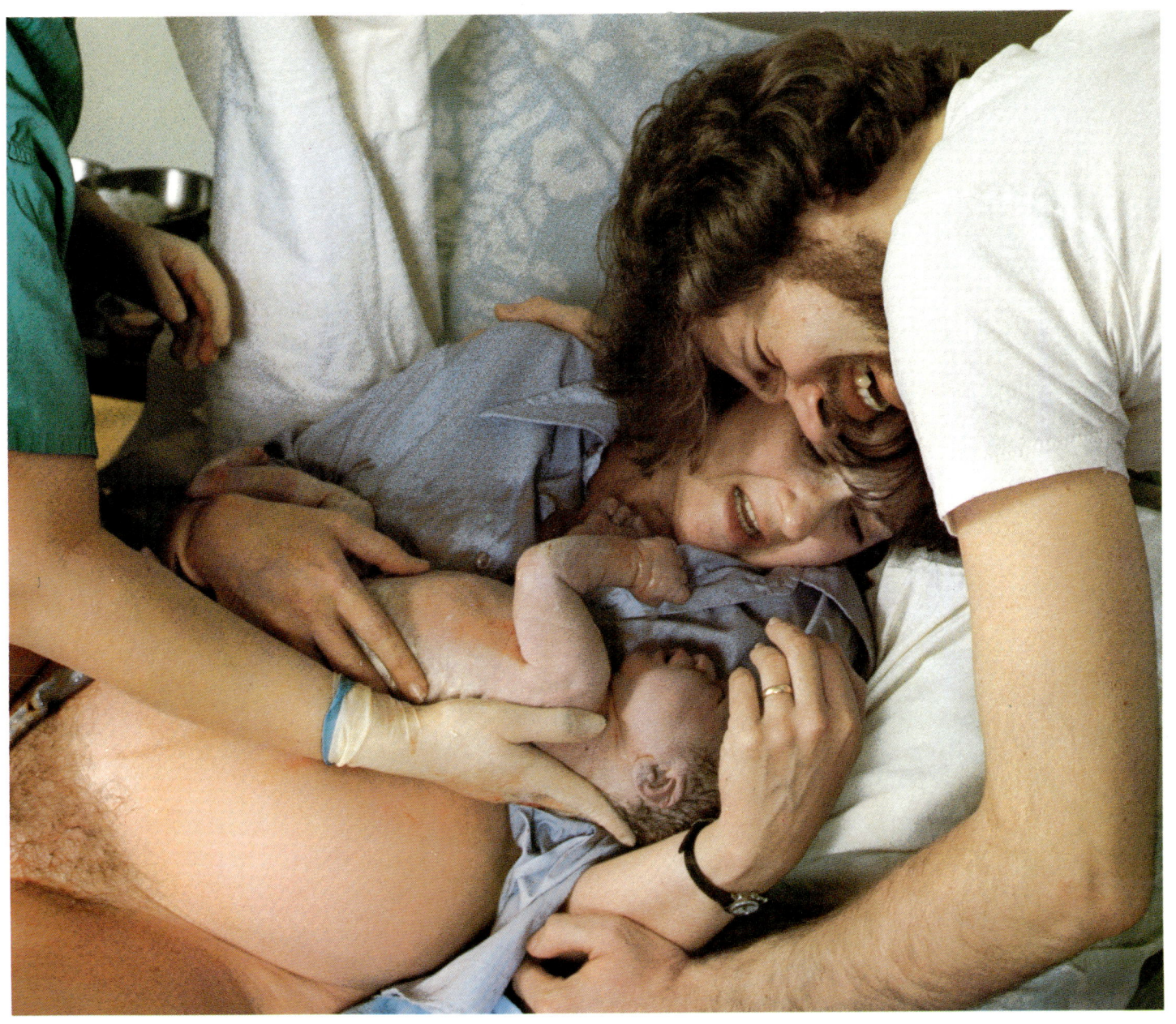

David: I didn't even try to stop my tears. This was the most profound sense of joy and relief I've ever felt about anything. Certainly this was the most powerful and emotional experience I've ever had.

Susan: I've never been happier! I told the midwives that I felt like I owed them my life.

David: It wasn't until about ten minutes later that we found out our baby was a boy. We were all so busy rejoicing that he was finally here that nobody even thought to look!

Susan and I hadn't settled on a boy's name beforehand, and we still had a problem choosing among several. Finally I just said, "Well, then, let's name him Douglas." Susan agreed, and I remember thinking that was a very arbitrary way to make a decision that he'll have to live with for the rest of his life.

Elongation of the baby's head

The skull bones of a baby are soft, and not closely knit together. They mold as the baby passes through the birth canal. This is why some babies have an elongated head at birth. The extent of the elongation depends on several factors: the size of the baby's head, the size of the mother's pelvis, the position of the baby, and, probably most important, the length of time the baby is in the birth canal. The head will resume a normal shape within twelve to seventy-two hours.

Susan had a particularly long labor; therefore, the baby was in the birth canal longer than usual. Because of this, the infant's bluish-gray color is more pronounced than it might be in babies who have gone through a shorter labor. This is only temporary, and as you will see, the baby soon turns a healthy pink color.

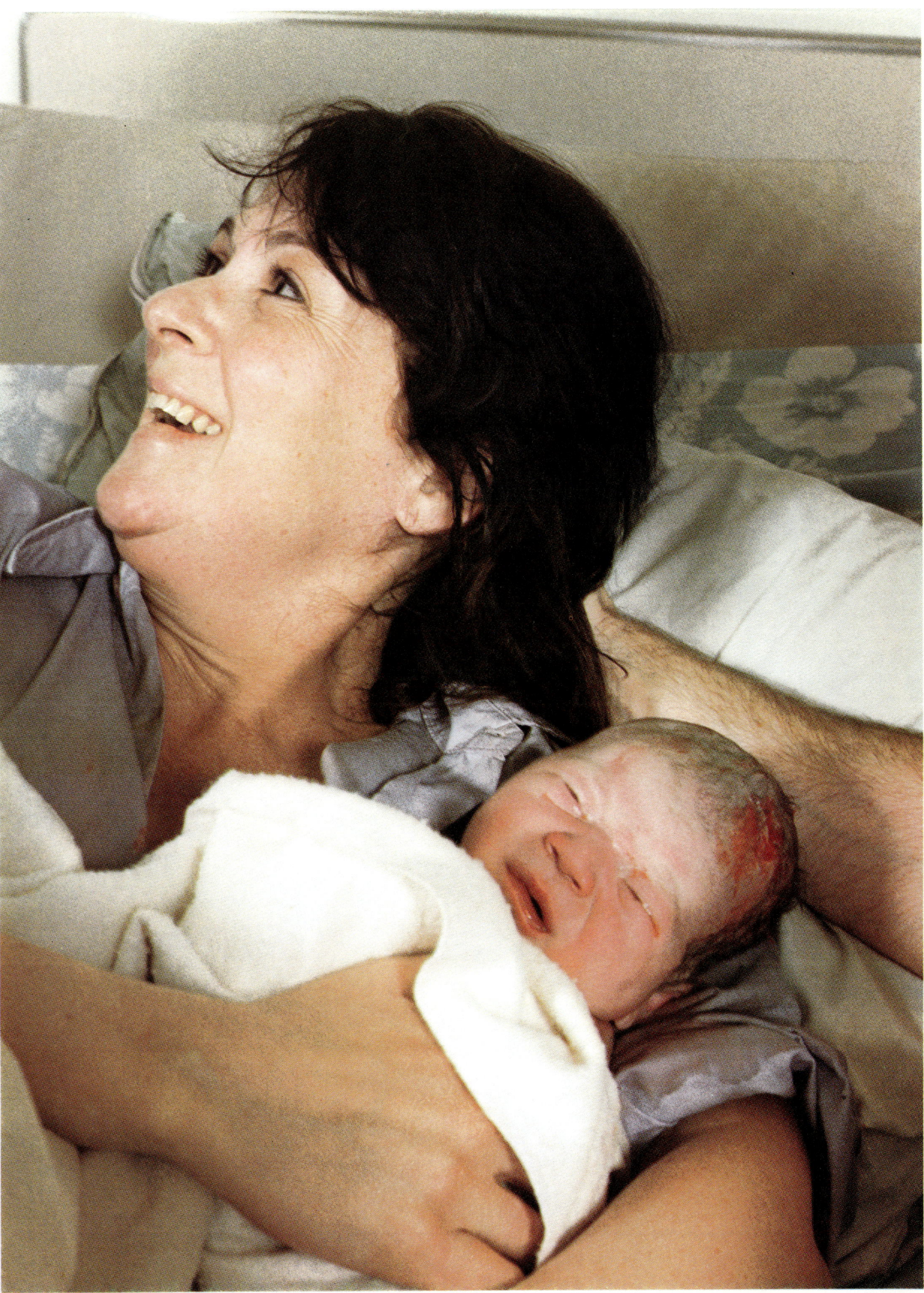

Susan: I wanted to try nursing him. He started sucking right away, and it was exhilarating to see that it really worked!

Nursing the baby immediately after birth
The baby's sucking will cause uterine contractions, which will help with the involution of the uterus to its original size. This process may take up to two weeks, and the mother will notice that each time she nurses her baby, her uterus contracts.

Also, putting the baby to the breast immediately will help the mother to bond with it. The touching of the skin is important, even if the baby is not interested in nursing yet.

The mother will have only colostrum at the beginning. The baby is not getting any milk yet. However, colostrum is exactly the right nourishment for a newborn. It is a light, protein-rich fluid that is easy to digest. It will also give the baby the mother's immunities. So it is advisable that the mother not wait until her milk comes in before she nurses her baby. Also, stimulating the breasts will make the milk come in sooner.

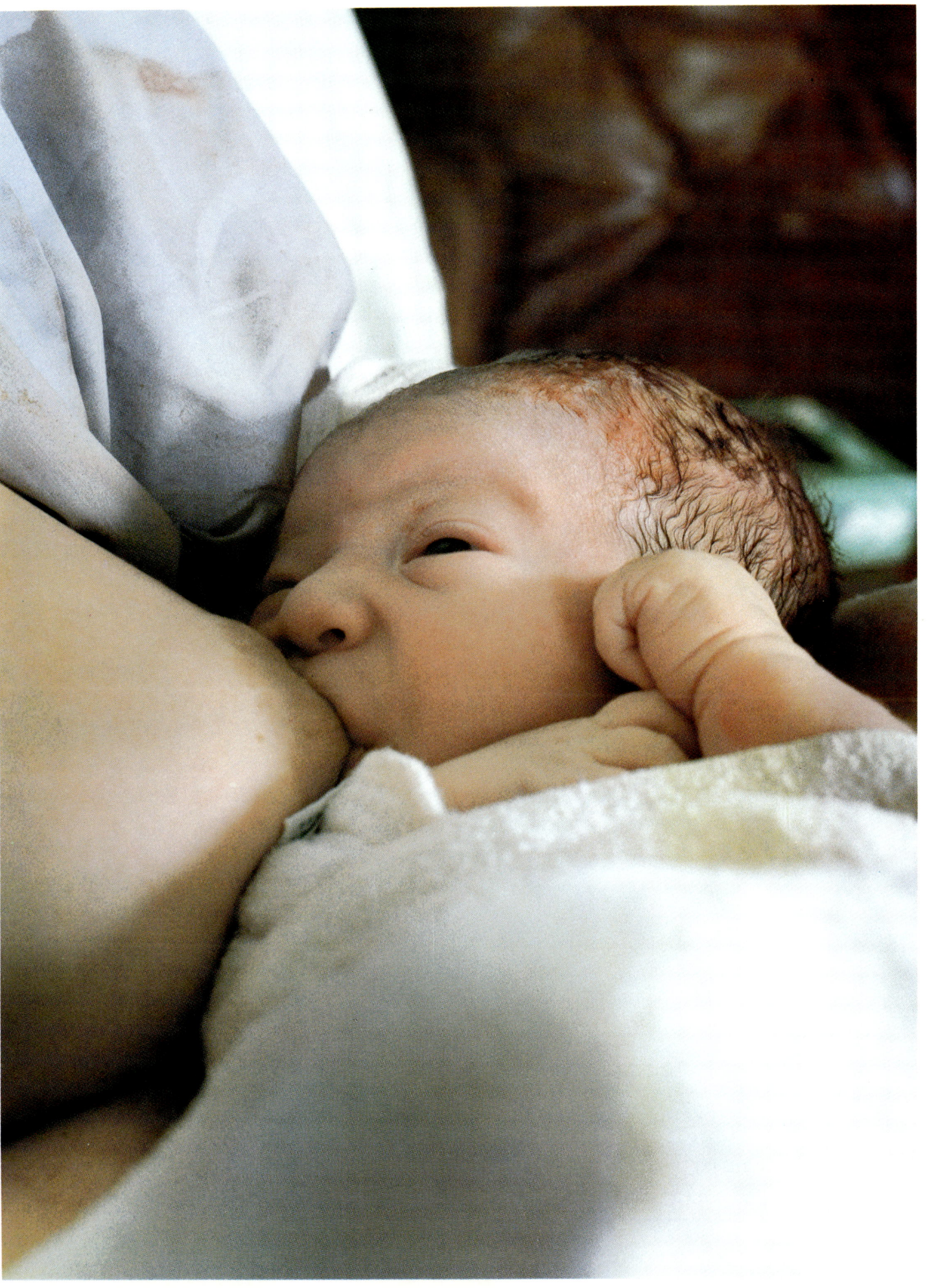

Susan: I was really glad that David was this close to me. His head was touching mine, and he was holding me. I think that we were probably more in love here than we have ever been.

David: Yes, this was definitely the high point of our lives.

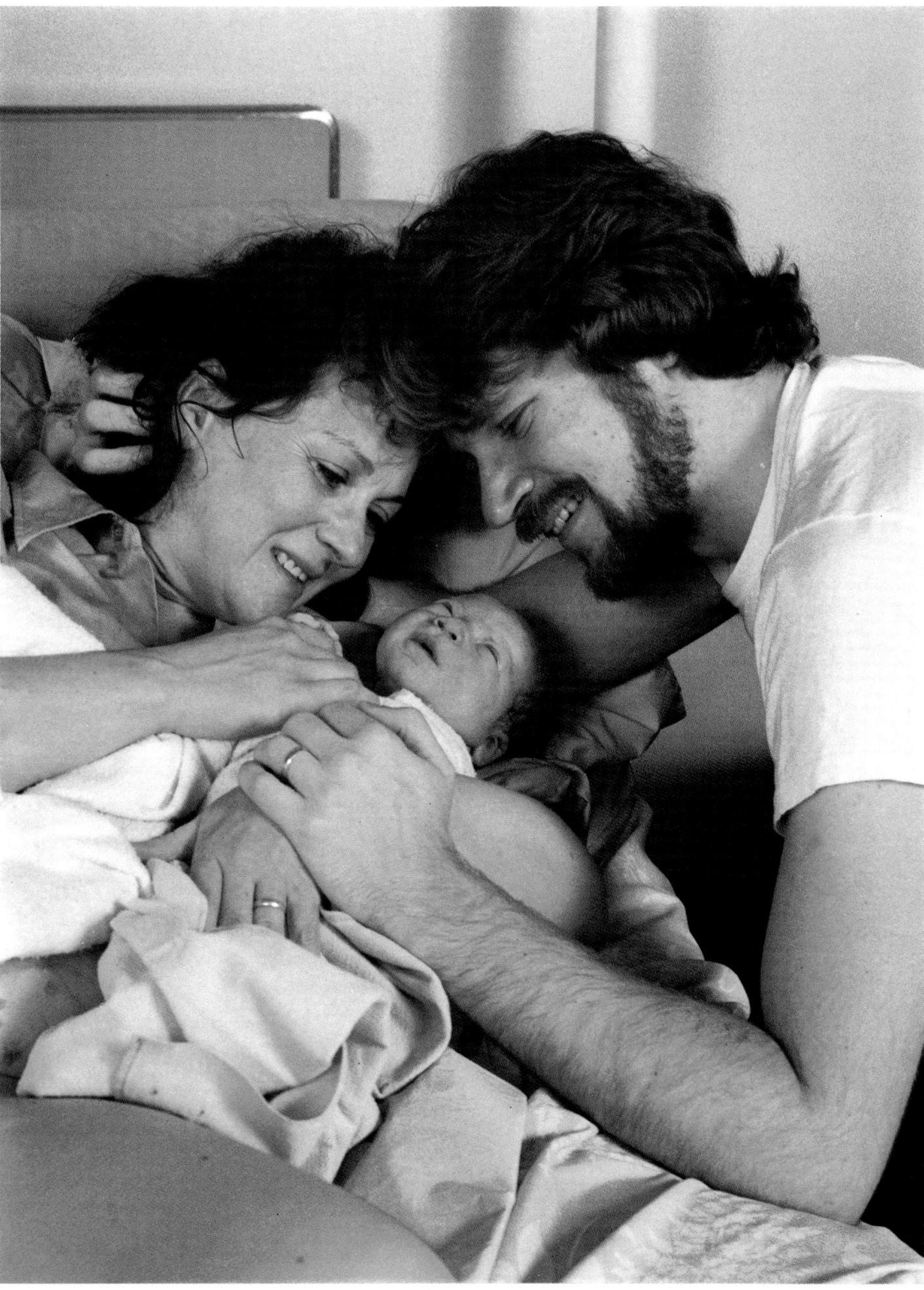

NANCY
·and·
TOM

Nancy: Even before I became pregnant again, Tom and I both knew that we would want our daughter, Kate, to be with us for the birth of her sibling. We had seen studies that showed the many benefits of having an older child present for the birth, but studies aside, it just seemed like the best thing for all of us. As soon as we knew for sure that I was pregnant, we began preparing her for the event.

Tom: I think most children, especially those as young as Kate, are likely to feel some kind of resentment toward a new sibling. This situation is aggravated when the mother leaves the child and disappears for days, returning with a new baby in her arms. Kate would be only two and a half when the new baby arrived, and Nancy and I both felt that if she were included, there would be much less cause for jealousy. The good feelings that she would have about being part of the birth would provide a positive basis for her relationship with the new baby.

Nancy: Right from the start, whenever we talked about the new baby, we always called it "our baby," meaning Kate's as well. She came with me for all my checkups, felt the baby move, and listened to its heartbeat. We looked at pictures that showed fetal development, and I explained that our baby looked a lot like the ones in the photographs. I think that all of this helped Kate develop some sort of an attachment to the baby. Certainly she was excited about it.

During the last months of my pregnancy, we started making plans for the actual birth. Kate would need a "support person," that is, someone who would take care of all her needs, both physical and emotional. My sister, Kathleen, and I have always been close, and I knew that if she were there, it would be nice for me as well as for Kate. At the same time that Kathleen would be a big help to us, I felt she would get a lot out of being the support person. I think giving birth is one of the most intimate times in life. In asking Kathleen to be present, I was able to tell her in a very special way how much I love her.

Kathleen: I felt proud that Nancy asked me to be Kate's support person. She explained what was involved, and I was determined to meet the responsibility as best I could. More so than for myself, I wanted the birth to be very special for Kate. After all, it was her baby brother or sister who was coming into the world. I began to prepare myself so that I could be as helpful to her as possible when the time came. We read books together that explained what would be happening. I thought about the different situations that might arise, as well as the questions that Kate might ask.

I was very excited that I was going to be there when my sister gave birth, and I couldn't wait for it to happen. I loved telling my friends about it, although most of them were quite surprised and didn't know what to say.

Tom: With all the plans set, it was just a matter of waiting for the big day.

Nancy: Early that morning, I started having contractions. Tommy and I discussed whether or not he should go to work, or if he did how quickly he could get back. By eight A.M. the contractions were coming regularly, and we knew for sure that I was in labor. Kathleen was easy to reach, and she said she'd meet us at the Maternity Center.

I had thought a lot about how I was going to conduct myself this time, and I really wanted to be super calm and collected throughout the entire labor. There were many things that I had wanted to do the first time around and never got a chance to. This morning I took a shower, washed my hair, blew it dry, and even put on makeup, stopping now and then to do my breathing. Tommy went to get the car while I packed some food for the family.

Tom: In the beginning of the labor, I was very worried. Kate's birth had been really hard on Nancy. Kate was very big, and posterior. Nancy had severe back labor, and it dragged on. The contractions kept coming, and she rarely had a rest period. It was still a normal delivery, but it was just difficult. I was concerned that the same thing was going to happen again. I reminded myself that Nancy and I were much more prepared this time around, and that this was Nancy's second baby would surely make things easier.

Posterior presentation

In a posterior presentation, the baby starts out facing the mother's belly, so that the back of its head is pressed against her spine. Generally this slows down the labor and frequently causes the mother pain in her back. Also the baby's head will have to be rotated 180 degrees while the mother is pushing so that the infant can face her spine and then pivot as it emerges to look straight into the world at birth. This often causes the second stage of labor, the expulsion stage, to be longer and more painful than usual. Occasionally it may require some help from the midwife or doctor.

Tom: Driving on the F.D.R. was difficult, to say the least. It was during the morning rush hour, which didn't help, but worse were the bumps in the road. Nancy's contractions were fairly strong by now, and driving over those bumps was very painful for her. Several times, I actually had to stop the car. I was quite relieved when we got there.

Nancy: Because I had given birth to Kate at the Center, it was like a second home to me. Kathleen was already there and helped Kate get settled. I got undressed, and Linda, the midwife, examined me.

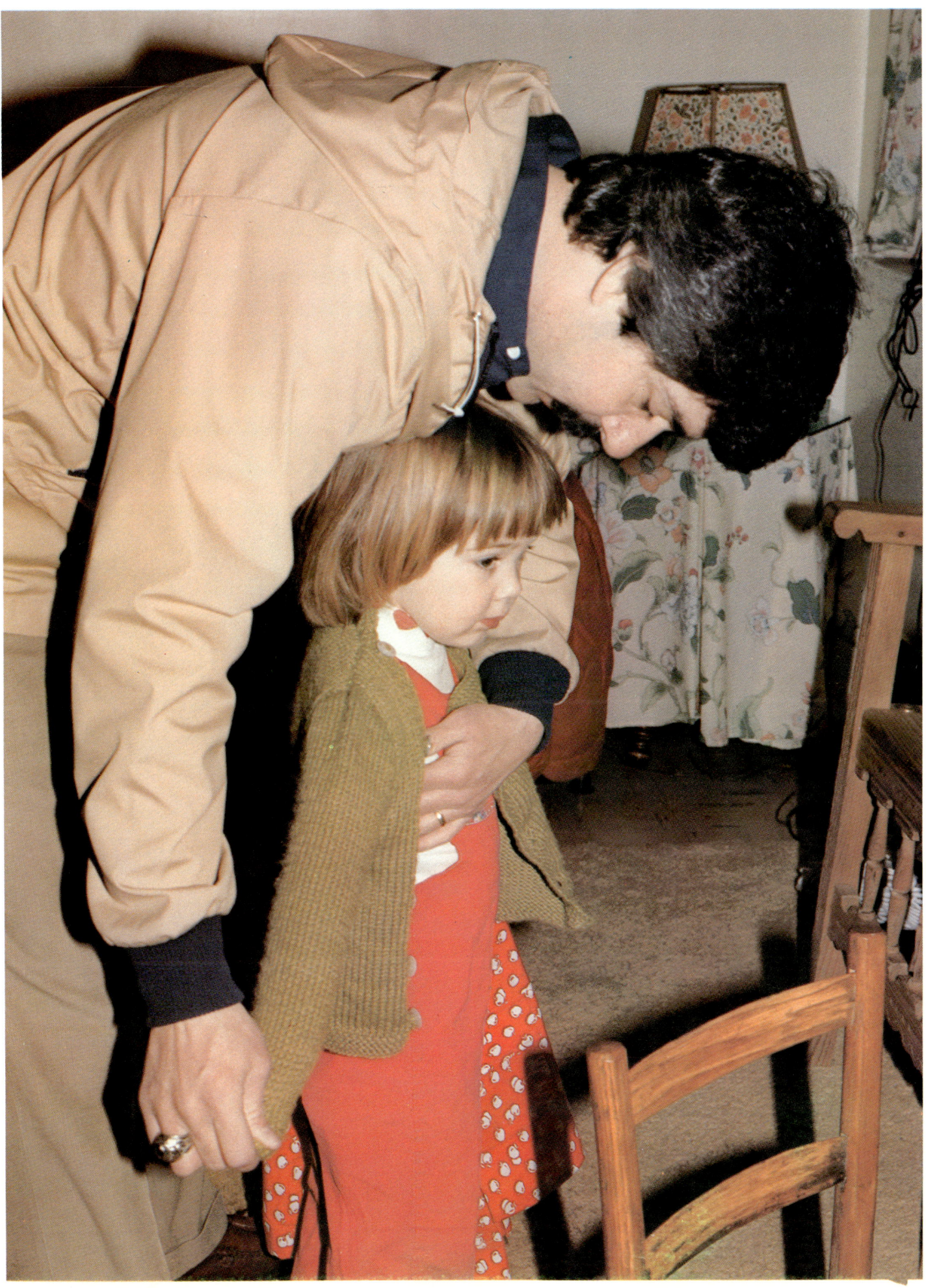

Nancy: Linda was a real doll! She was exactly what I needed for that birth. After evaluating my needs, she realized that I was happiest just being with my family and in control of the situation. I wanted to feel like I was running the show for as long as possible. She didn't hover over me, but I knew that anytime I needed her she would stay with me for as long as I wanted.

Linda checked the baby's heartbeat many times throughout the labor, and, as I explained to Kate, it's always reassuring to hear that things are fine.

Having Kate there was really helpful, especially when labor became difficult. I might be having terrifically painful contractions, but there was Kate, watching *Sesame Street* and eating yogurt. Watching her took my mind off things and brought me back to earth. She carried on with her everyday activities, and the sense of normalcy she provided helped me remain calm.

Kathleen was also an extra source of emotional support. She was wonderful with Kate, but also it was nice talking to her and just knowing she was there.

Tom: By now, I was feeling great! Everything was going so well. If we could have planned the labor to go exactly as we wanted it to, things couldn't have been much better.

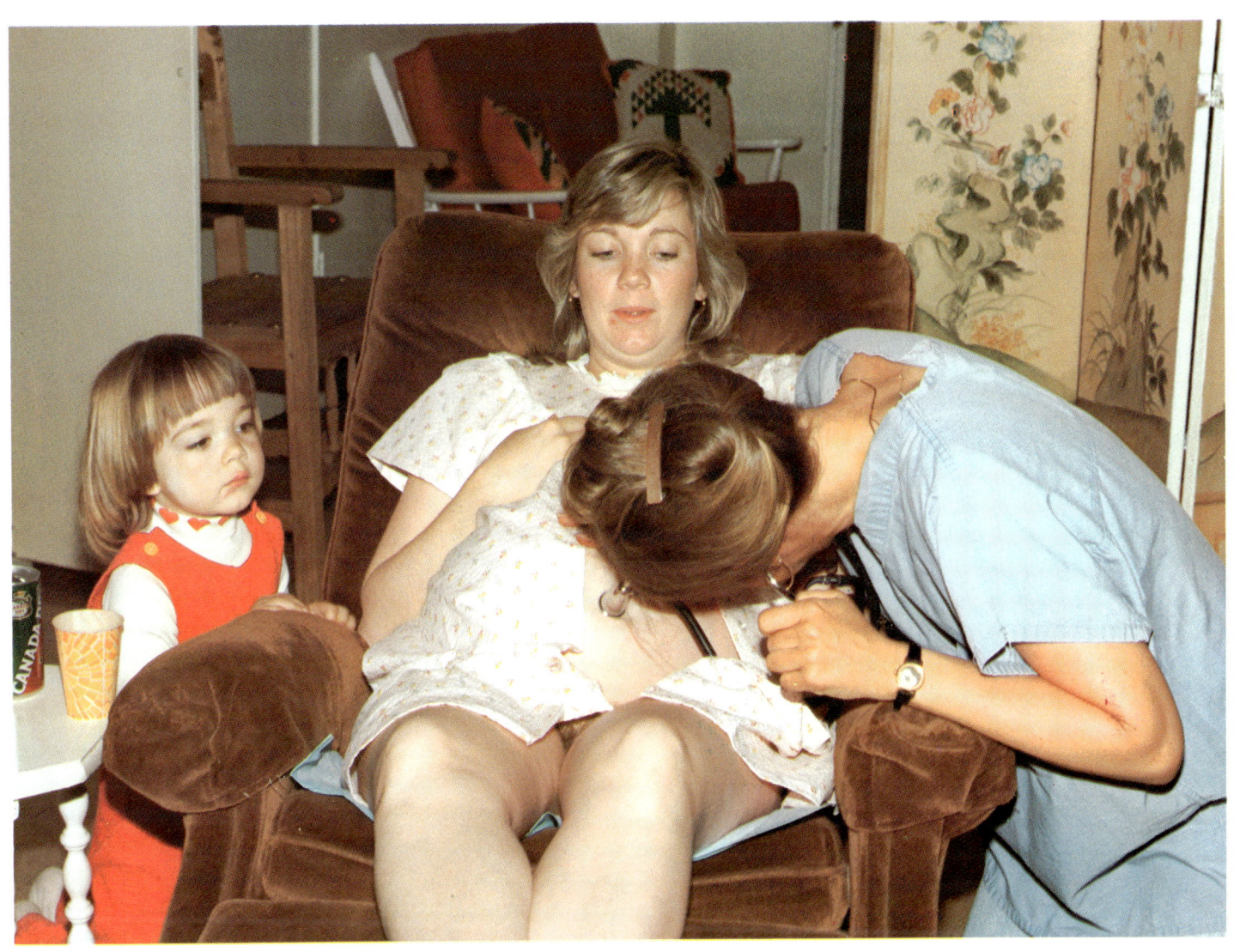

The fetal heart is checked continuously
It is extremely important that the midwife or doctor keep in close touch with the baby to know how it is faring during the hours of labor and strenuous contractions. Each contraction of the uterus somewhat cuts down the oxygen supply to the baby. This is a normal occurrence, but it is important to know that the baby has gotten back its full supply of oxygen immediately after the contraction. Therefore, the attendants frequently check the fetal heart either by attaching a fetal monitor to the mother's abdomen, which measures the strength of the contractions as well as indicating the frequency of the fetal heartbeat, or through continuous listening with a special stethoscope, or fetoscope.

The fetal heart rate is much more frequent than an adult's heart rate. A rate between 120 and 160 beats per minute is considered normal in a fetus, whereas an adult will have only between sixty and ninety beats per minute.

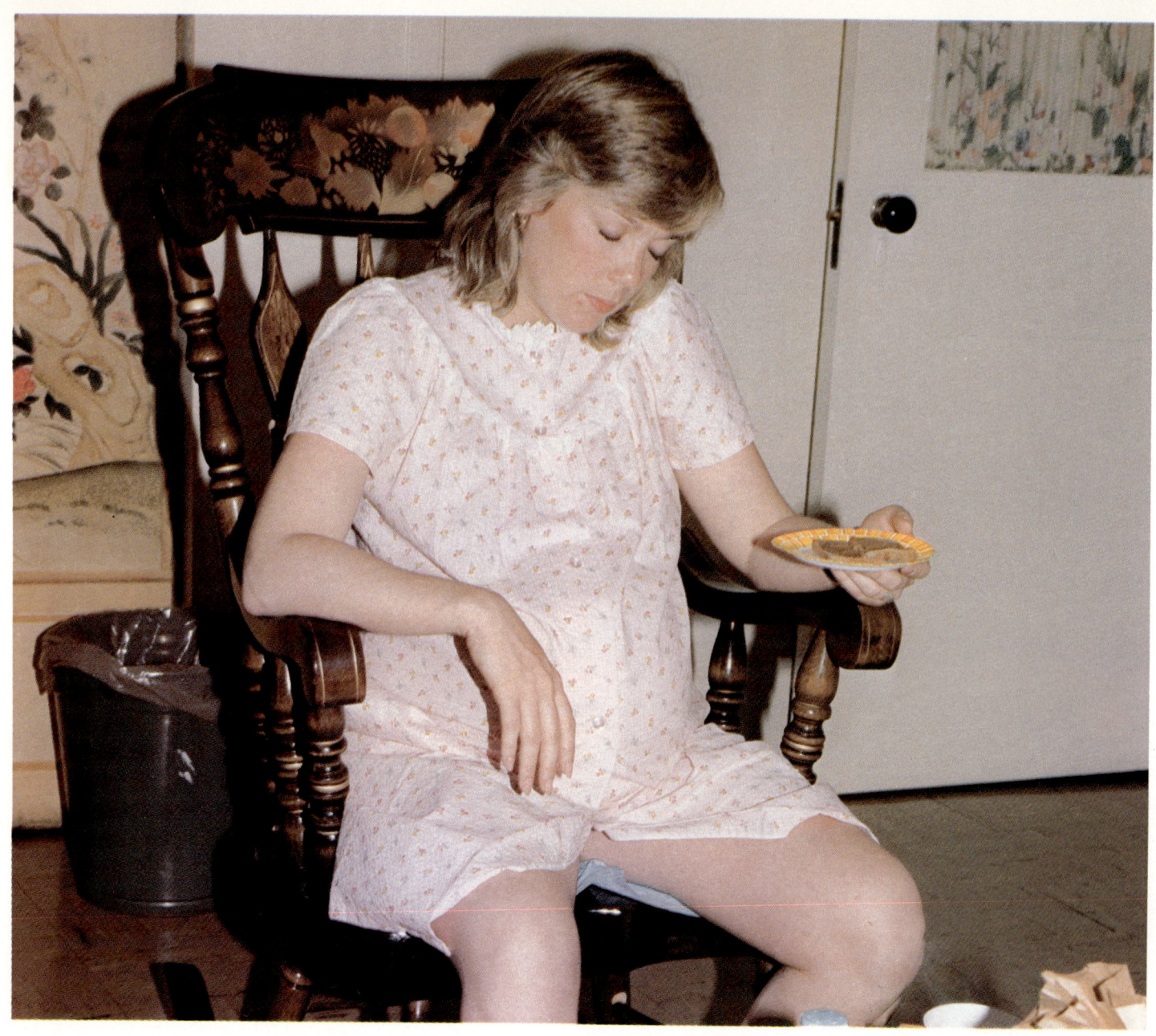

Nancy: I hadn't had anything to eat yet that morning, so I went and got a piece of toast. As soon as I sat down again, another contraction came on. I knew that maximum relaxation was important. I let most of my extremities go limp, but I wasn't going to drop that piece of toast! I was so hungry.

Lamaze relaxation techniques
These techniques help a woman become so aware of her body that she can deliberately relax parts of it while other parts are in tension and working. One of the great advantages of being able to relax during contractions is that it will help reduce pain in labor. It will also allow the woman to work with her body instead of against it, and to ride the contractions smoothly instead of being thrown by them. It is a difficult thing to learn, and demands practice and absolute concentration on her part.

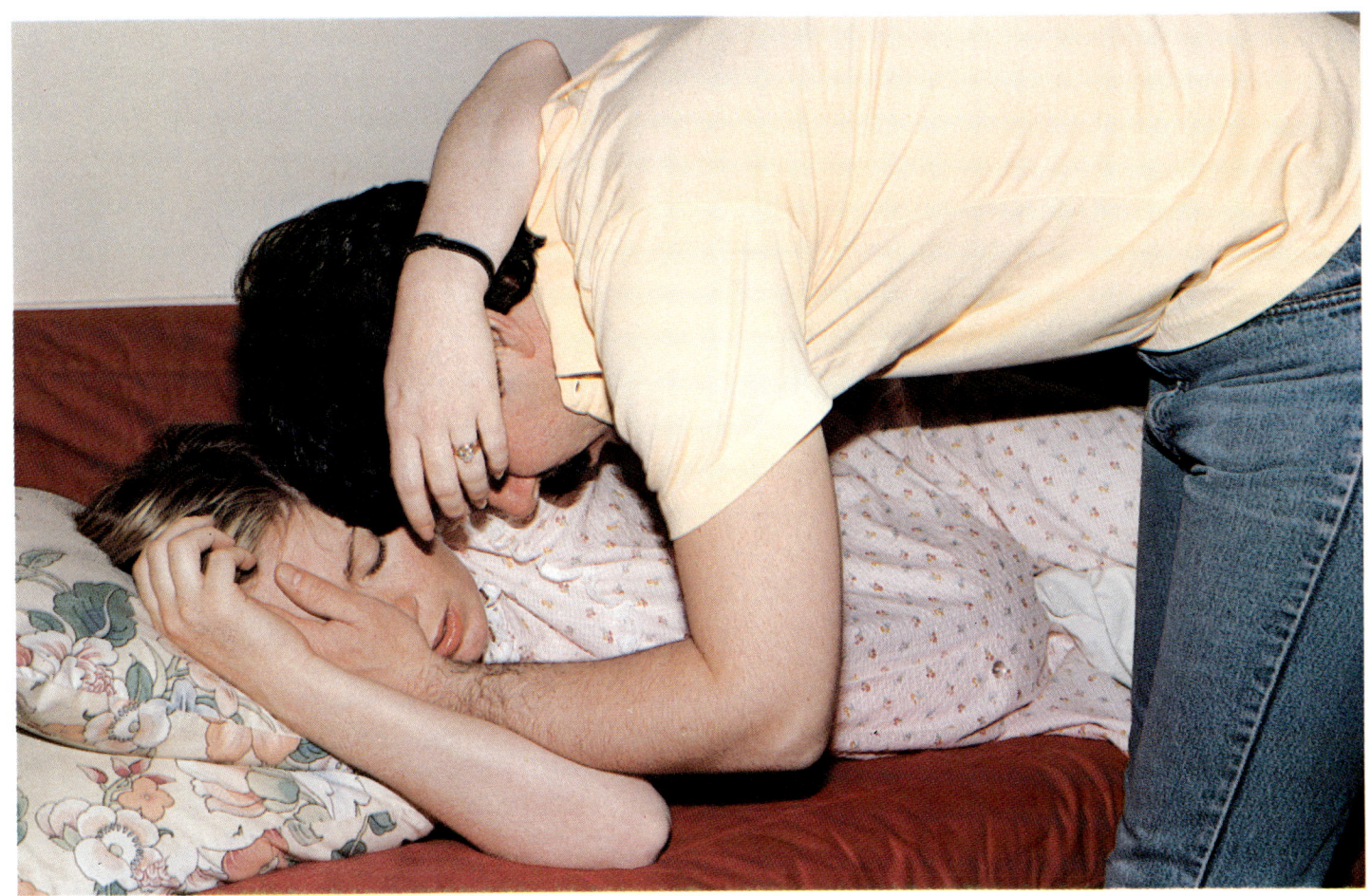

Tom: I was able to follow exactly where Nancy was in her labor just by the way she was acting. During the past few hours, when she wasn't having a contraction, we were talking and even laughing. But once transition hit, her whole disposition changed. There was no more laughter, just hard work.

Nancy: Things were getting rough, and I remember thinking, "I hope I can make it through without losing control." Then I said to myself, "Take it one contraction at a time. Just get through this one and worry about the coming contractions later."

I tried to occupy myself with the television, but Kate was a better distraction. She came over and started talking to me. I remember that she made me smile, which was not easy during transition.

Tom: Anytime she did smile, even briefly, I was overjoyed. I was glad to see that at least she was getting rest periods in between contractions.

It can be very frustrating to be the main support person. I could let Nancy squeeze my hand as hard as she needed to, even until it turned blue, but sometimes that wasn't enough. I wanted to do so much more for her, but I just couldn't share the pain.

Nancy: As the contractions increased in intensity, I would pull Tommy in tighter and tighter. I wanted desperately to crawl into his body. He had a comforting effect, and the closer he got to me, the better I felt.

Nancy: I was really listening to my body throughout the entire labor. I don't know what it was, but something inside me said, "It's time to go into the birthing room and do what you're here to do." It wasn't as if one contraction finally was more severe than the others, or that my membranes had ruptured. It was a natural thing, like a nesting instinct, that told me to settle down into the place where I knew my baby was to be born.

Tom: Just before she got onto the bed, she was hit with an extra-long contraction.

Nancy: Once again, Kate came to the rescue. She was so cute, helping me with my slippers, and the levity she provided lightened up a very serious moment.

Tom: She seemed very concerned here about being left out. She was right on our tails, determined to be helpful.

Nancy: The last contractions were the longest and most difficult. I had one that was like a double contraction. It started, peaked, and then began to subside. That's generally when I got a rest period, but all of a sudden, it peaked again. I thought, "Hey, that wasn't fair, two contractions without a break in between."

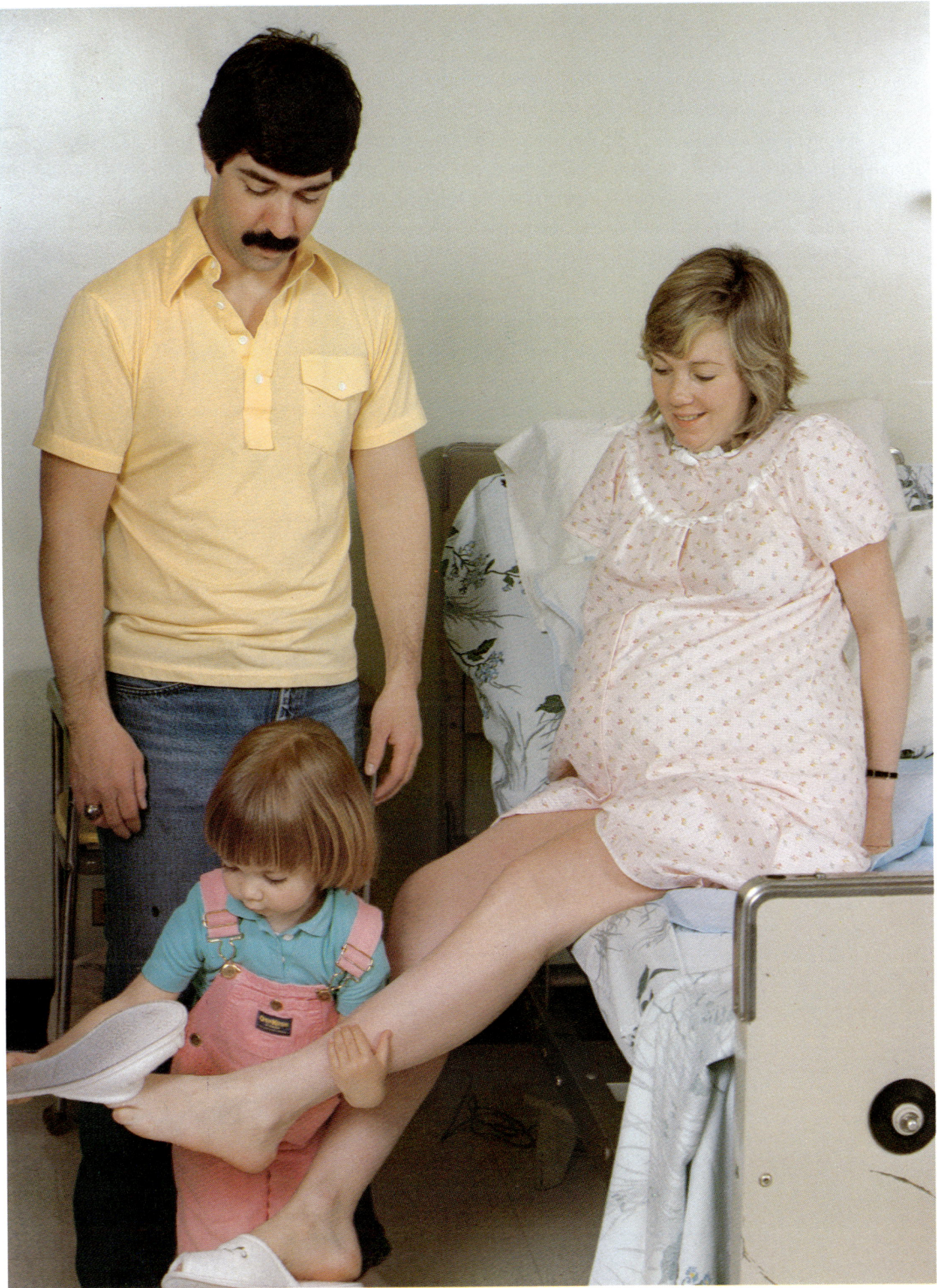

Nancy: Linda suggested that I deliver on my side, explaining that it would probably be easier and more comfortable for me. She said I was fully dilated now and should start pushing with the next contraction. I wanted to cooperate with everything she and Tom were telling me, when to push and when to pant. At this point, things were so intense that it was hard for me not to just draw into myself, but I managed to stay in tune with them.

My first push was very good, and it brought the baby right down. But the baby felt incredibly big, and as it was stretching its way out, it caused a terrible burning sensation. I began screaming and even though it did hurt, I knew at the time that the yelling was disproportionate to the amount of pain I was in. There was absolute chaos in the front part of my brain, but somewhere in the back of my mind I remember thinking, "Would you listen to yourself? You're screaming your head off! It's not that bad, so why are you doing this?" But then the other part of me thought, "So what? This is my birth, and I can make all the noise I want to." Childbirth educators say that if you yell, you expend your energy through your mouth, and aren't able to push as effectively. I'd heard this before, but at the time the yelling seemed like an inner source of strength that summoned up all my energy. I guess it was just something that I needed to do at the time. However, I was glad to see that Kathleen took Kate out of the room for that moment.

The side position for delivery
Although the side position is not commonly used, it can be very advantageous for delivery, especially if the baby presents posteriorly. The mother is often more comfortable on her side, with both legs bent, the lower leg resting on the bed and the other supported by her partner, the nurse, or the midwife. This position helps keep the pelvic muscles, including the perineum, relaxed, thus allowing the baby's head to emerge more easily. The mother manages well on her side, the midwife and her partner helping and encouraging her.

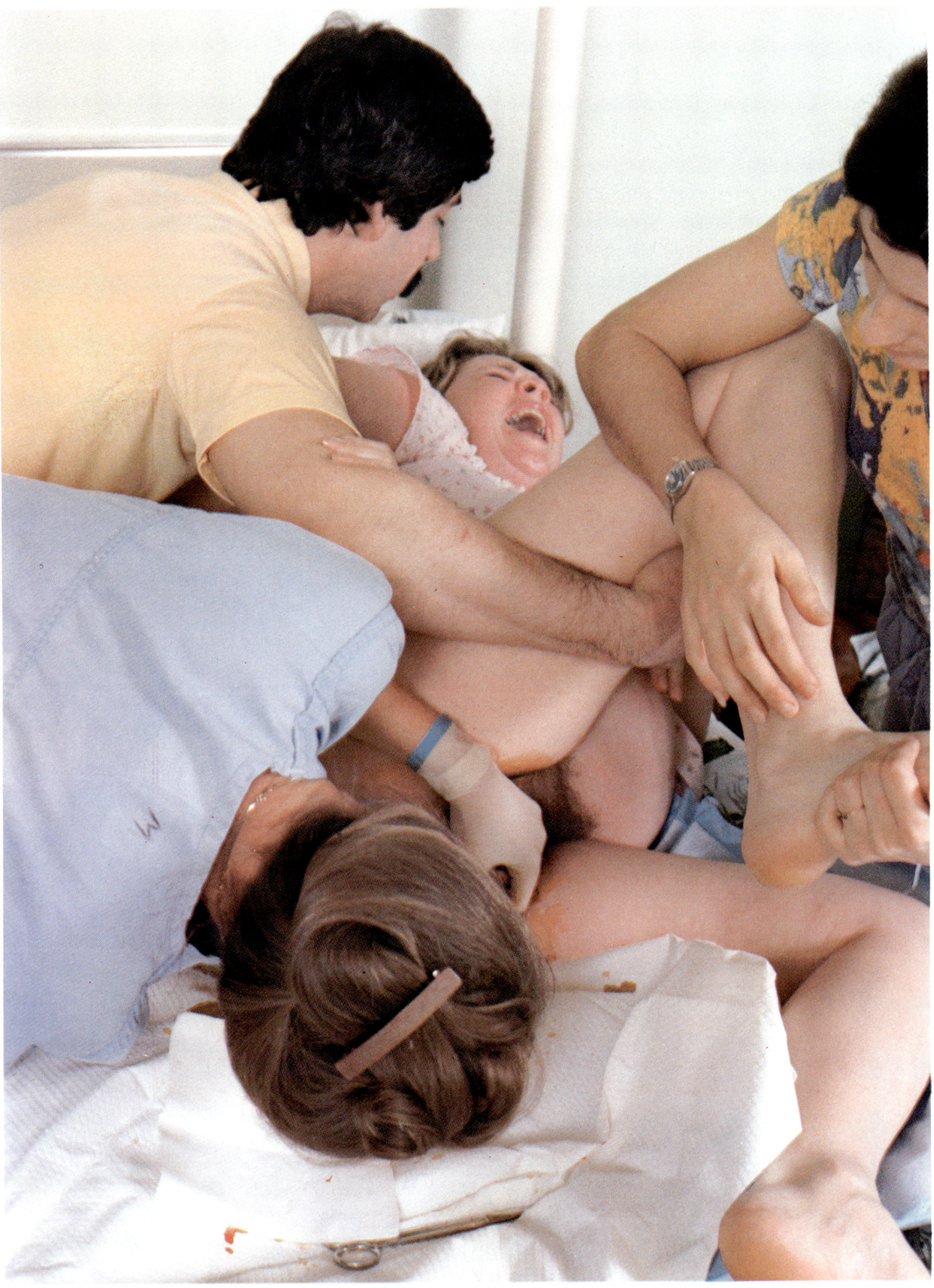

Nancy: The baby felt enormous, and I was sure I was going to have to push for at least an hour or so. I thought, "How on earth am I going to keep this up?" and said out loud, "I can't! I can't do this!" Linda laughed and said, "What do you mean you can't? The baby's head is right here!" I was so shocked when she said that. It all happened so fast I wasn't sure what she was talking about. I asked, "Here? Where? What do you mean the baby's head is right here?" Then I reached down to feel the baby. It was the greatest pleasure when I touched my baby for the first time.

Tom: After the head was out, it seemed to me like a very long time before the rest of the body followed. I was beginning to worry, although I suppose there really wasn't any reason to.

Nancy: When Kate was born someone was holding a mirror, so I was able to see her coming out of me. To this day, I can still vividly see her face as she was emerging from my body. This time, because of the position I was in, I couldn't really see the baby being born, but for the rest of my life, I'm sure I will remember the sensation of the head against my leg. It was warm and wet and heavy, just resting on my leg. I knew it was my baby's head, and it felt so wonderful.

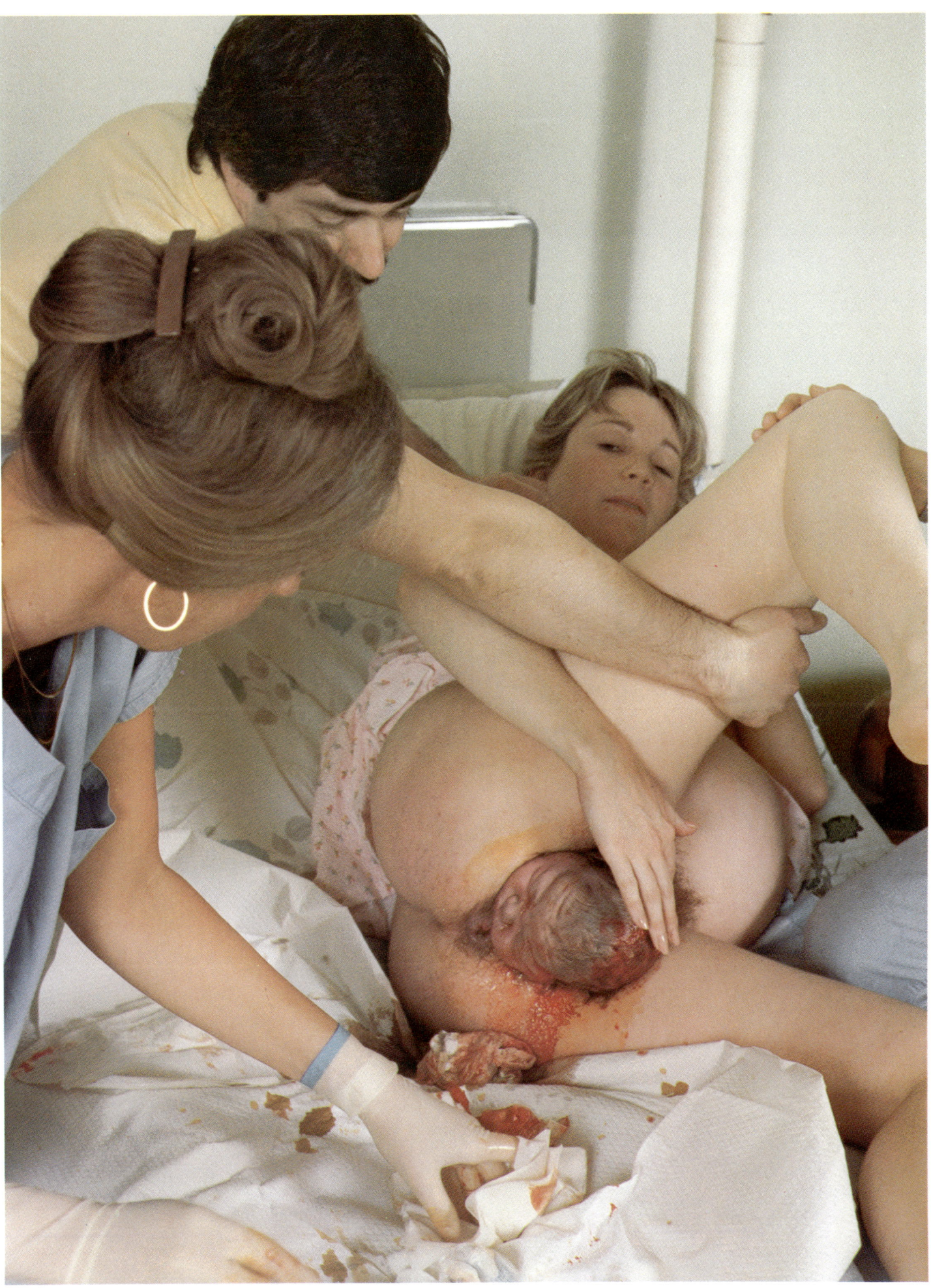

Tom: I was very fascinated by the baby, who was so close to me but not even completely born yet.

Nancy: I knew that everybody else was looking at the baby's face, but because of the position I was in, I couldn't see it. This was my baby, and I wanted to see it so badly. More than that, I desperately wanted to hold it.

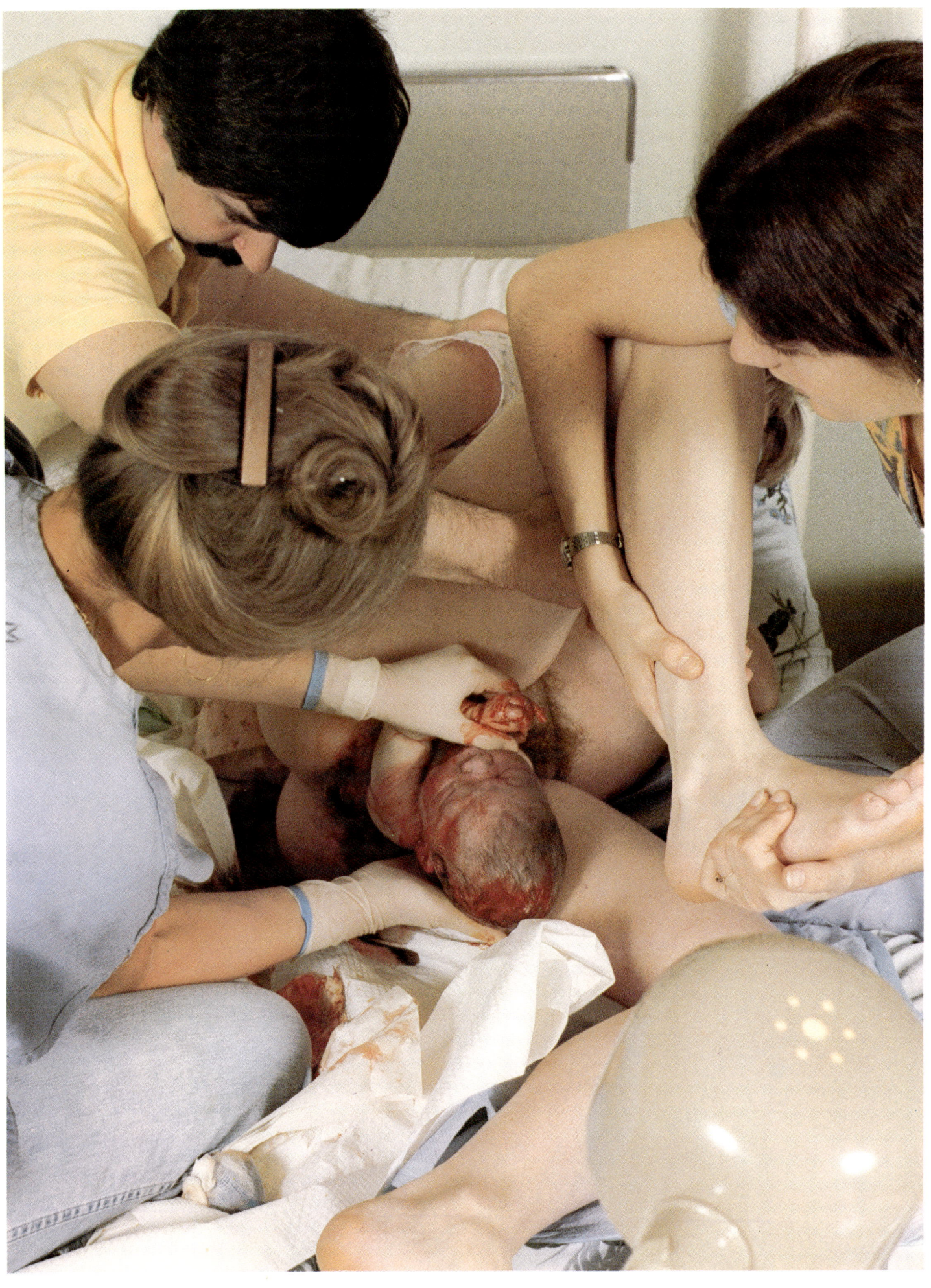

Nancy: I was so happy and overcome with emotion. I reached for the baby and, practically crying, I said, "I want to hold my baby!" I'd been waiting for this moment for so long, and now it was just seconds away!

Finally the baby was out, and in my arms!

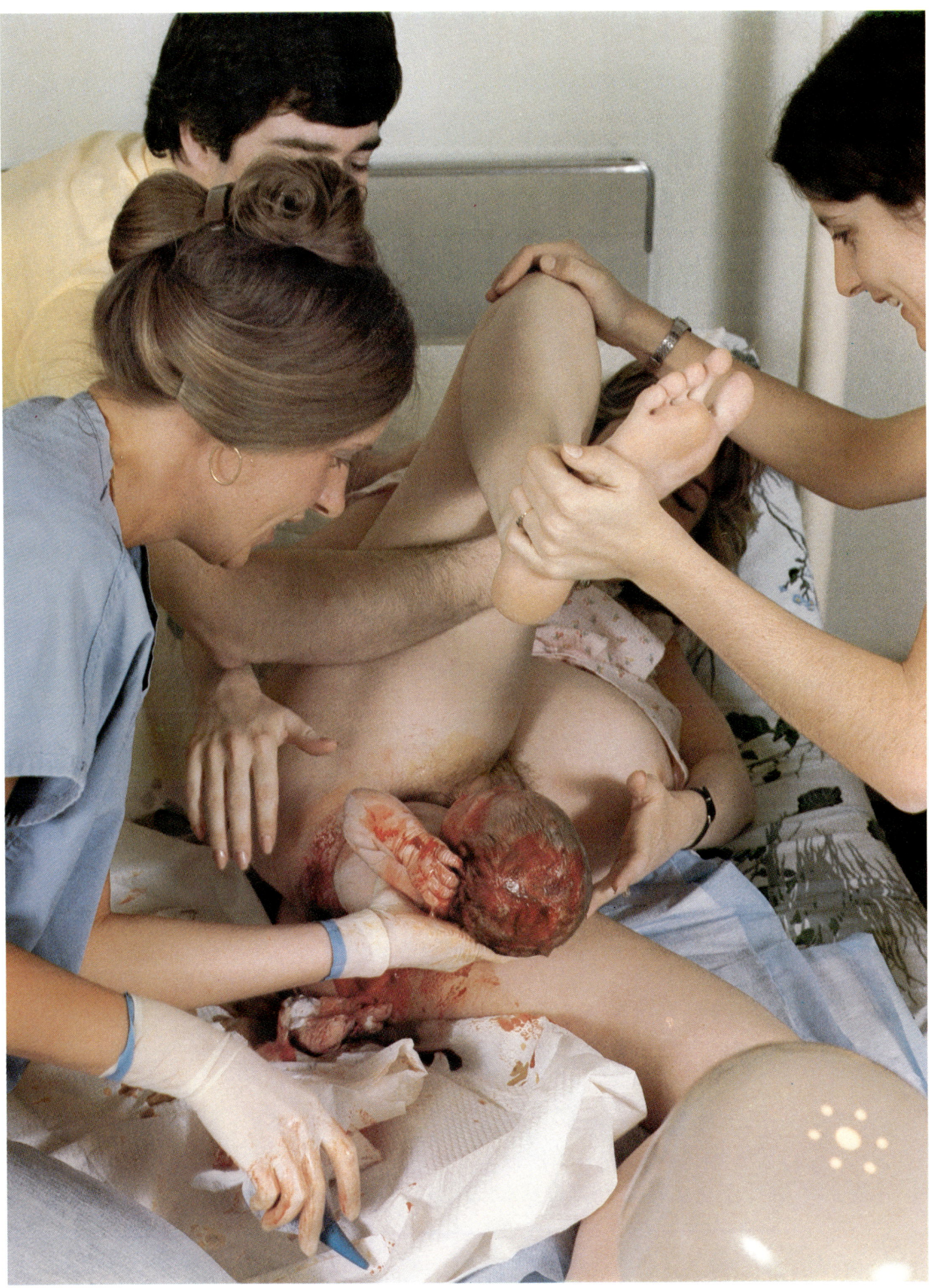

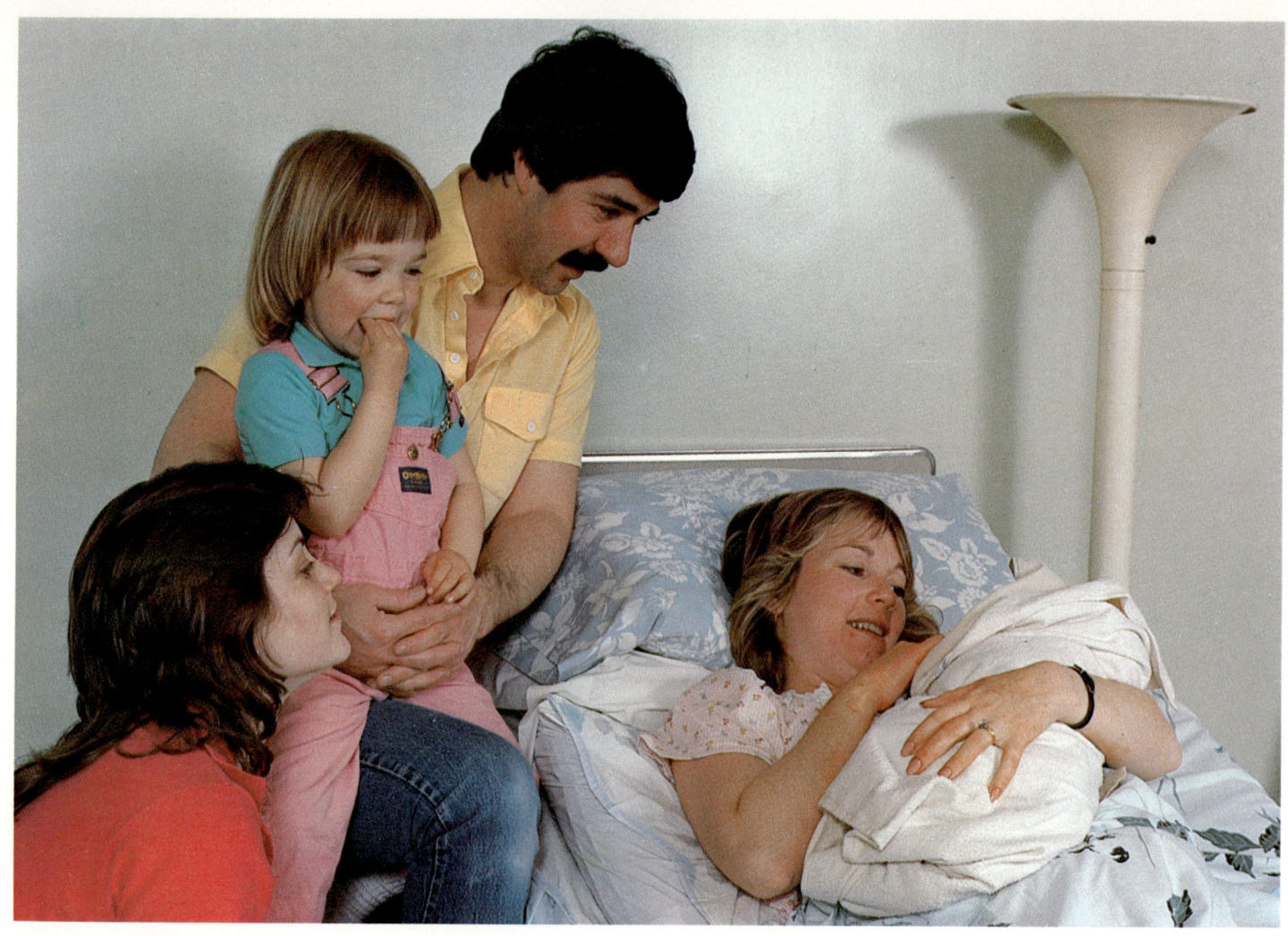

Tom: Kate giggled for about twenty minutes afterward. She was just so excited! Maybe she felt almost a little bit of disbelief. Even with all the preparation she'd had, she couldn't quite believe that he was really here at last. I guess it was pretty amazing for all of us.

Nancy: I was glad Kate was there the whole time, but even more so after Eric was born. Certainly there's nothing that's more of a family event than a birth, and I was so glad that we hadn't separated her from us.

Kathleen: I was in such awe of everything that was happening. I'd heard all these horror stories about giving birth, but this was all so warm and wonderful. I felt so lucky to be part of it.

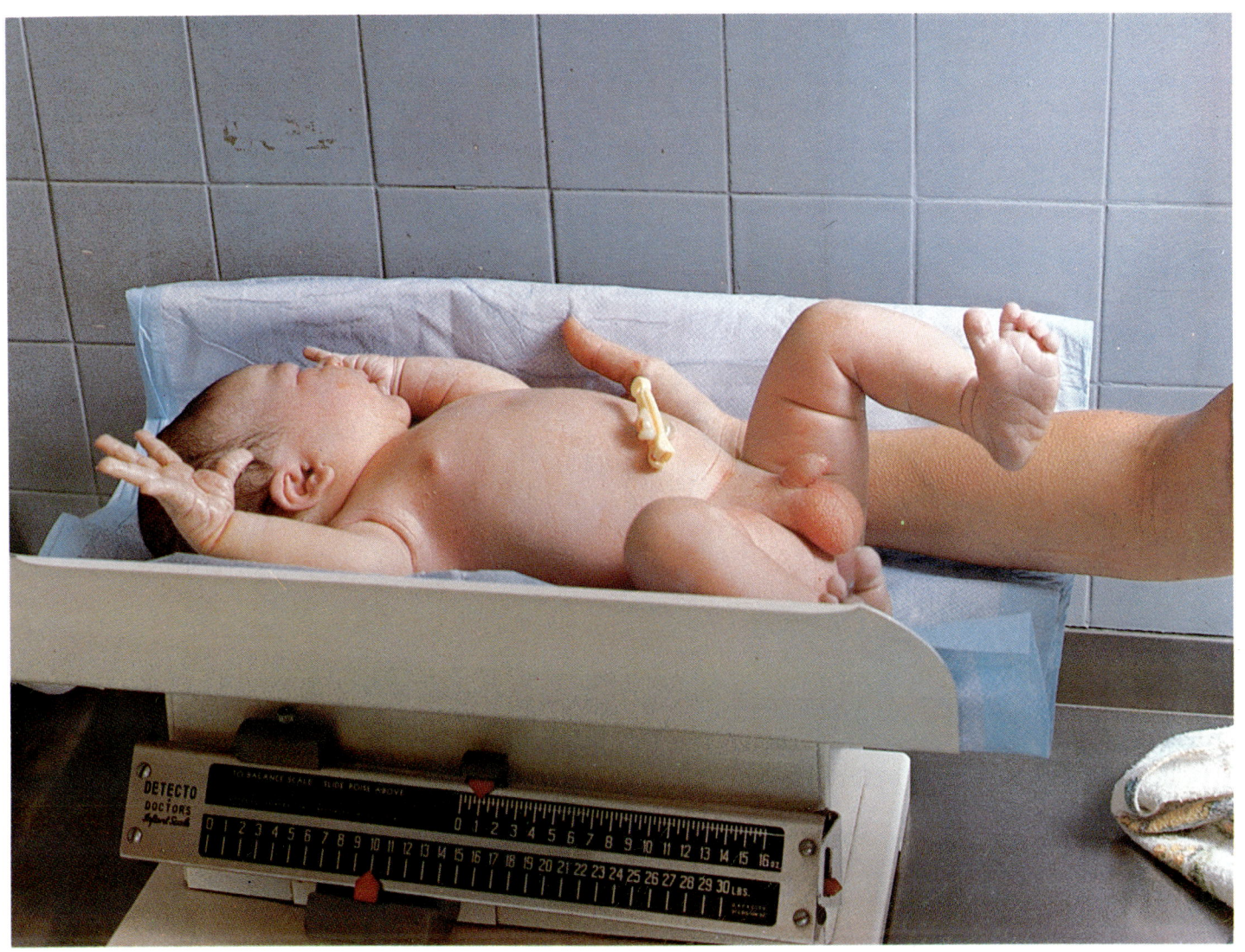

Tom: I was overjoyed! Almost as wonderful as having the new baby with us was the way we were able to conduct the labor and delivery. Nancy had done so magnificently, and I was thrilled about the entire event.

Nancy: I had known the baby was big, but when Linda said, "Ten pounds, one ounce," I couldn't believe it! No wonder it hurt to push him out!

Tom: I must say that I was quite shocked at having a boy. Unlike a lot of men, I had never felt any great need to have a son. Nancy and I have enjoyed Kate so much that we would have been very happy to have had another little girl. Not that we have created any sexist environment, but our life had been geared toward raising a daughter. So much so that I think we both almost assumed the new baby would be a girl. Admittedly, I was concerned about the differences there might be in raising a son, and I wondered about my own fathering abilities. I guess I was just having new-parent jitters though, because after a little time with my new son, it all felt right to me.

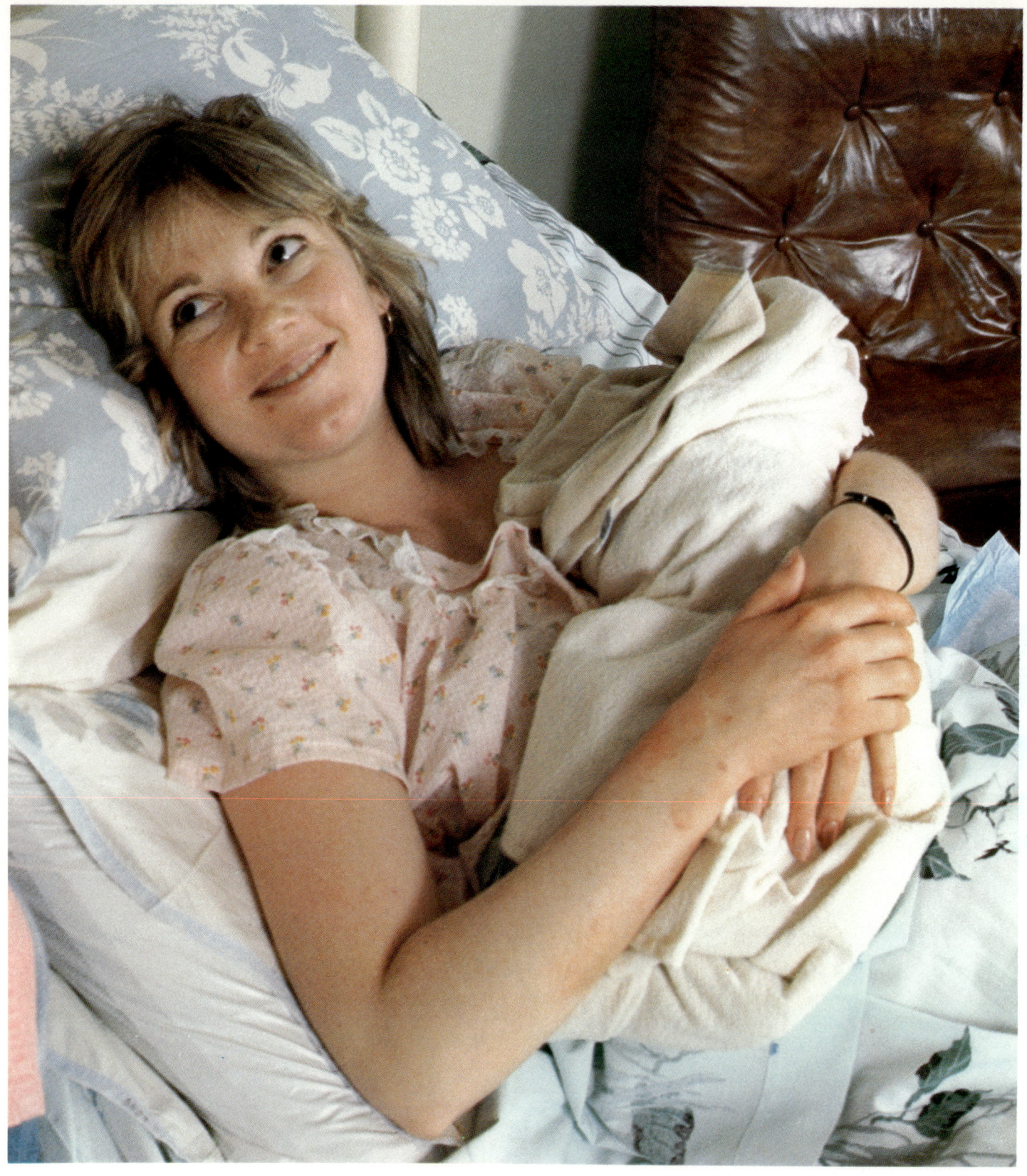

Nancy: Talk about emotional highs. Well, I was just floating on a cloud! Everything was so perfect.

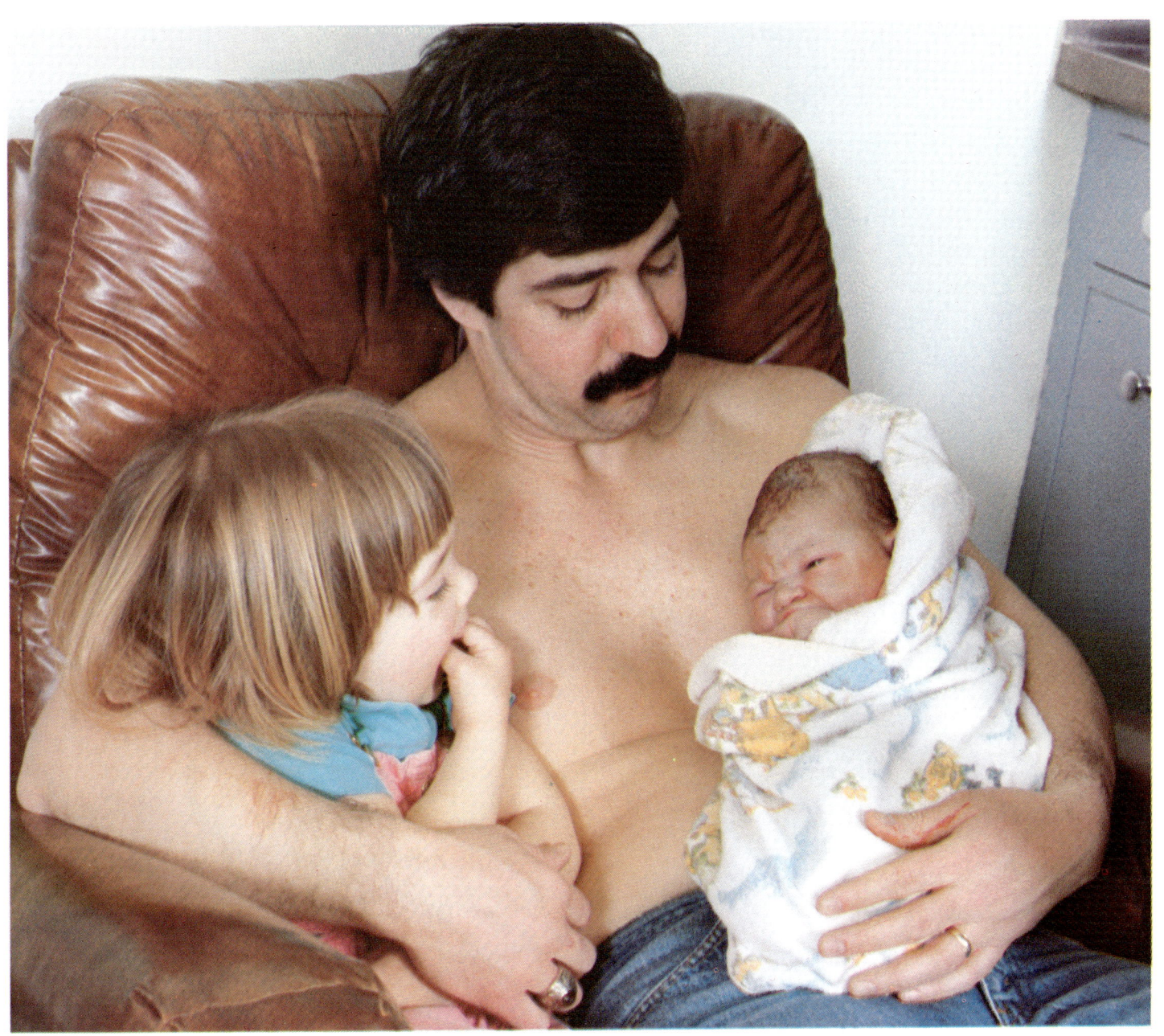

Tom: I wanted Kate to be included in the bonding with Eric. I took my shirt off so I could have skin-to-skin contact with my newborn, but the room wasn't that hot and he was all wrapped up. Kate seemed to be enjoying things just as they were, so I let it go until later. Besides, I was too happy to see past my two babies.

Nancy: I didn't want to push Eric on Kate. She's very young, and I wanted to give her a chance to accept him on her own terms. But she seemed thrilled about him right from the start, and I was so happy to see the way she responded to him.

A midwife came in to congratulate us, and Kate was proud to announce, "I was there when my baby brother was being born." It was clear that her involvement with the pregnancy and delivery made all the difference in the world with her feelings toward Eric.

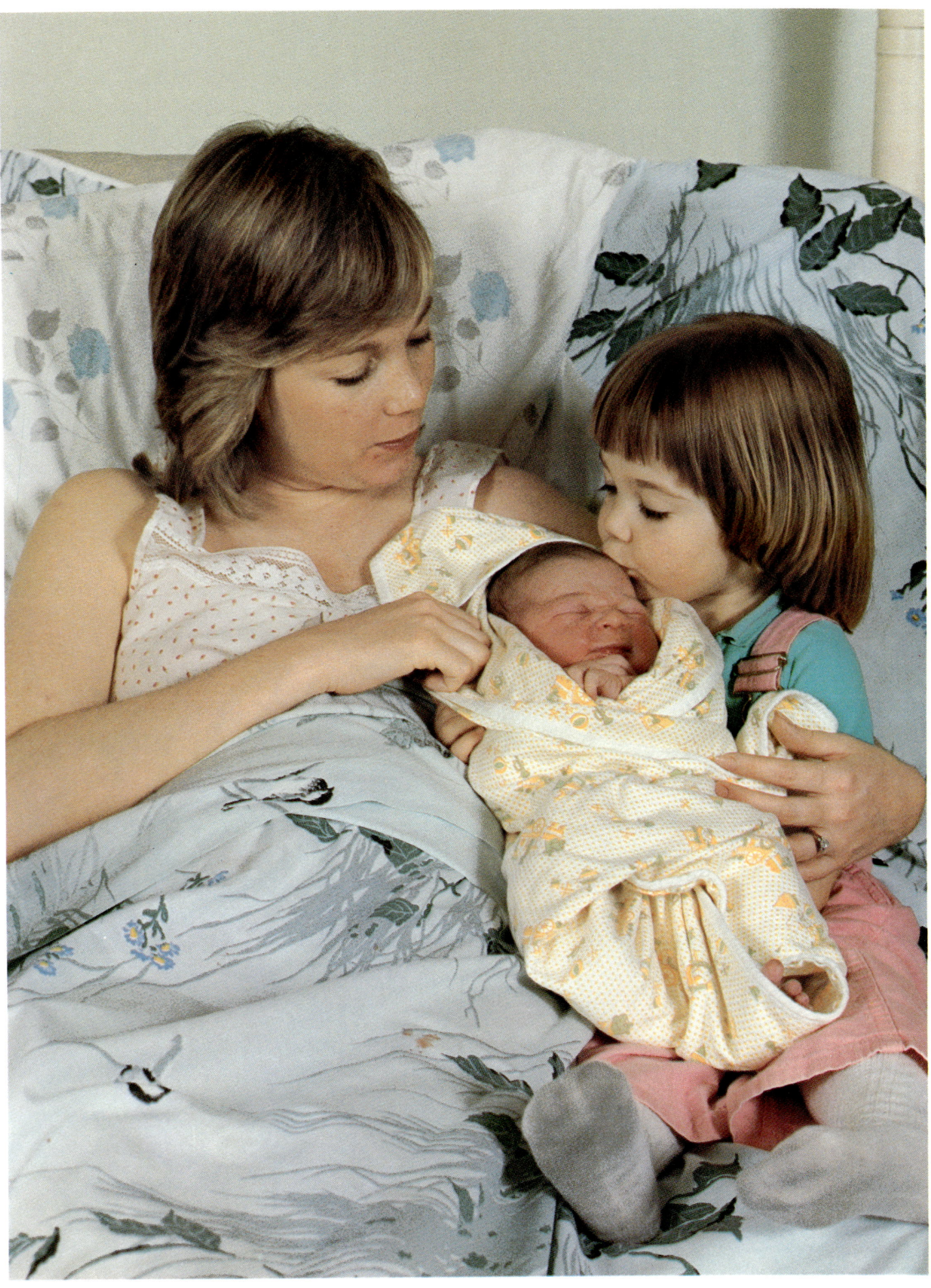

Nancy: Everyone had been helping me and giving me so much all day, and then of course when Eric was born, he was the center of attention. Therefore, it was very important to be alone here with Kate for a few minutes, just to hold her and cuddle with her.

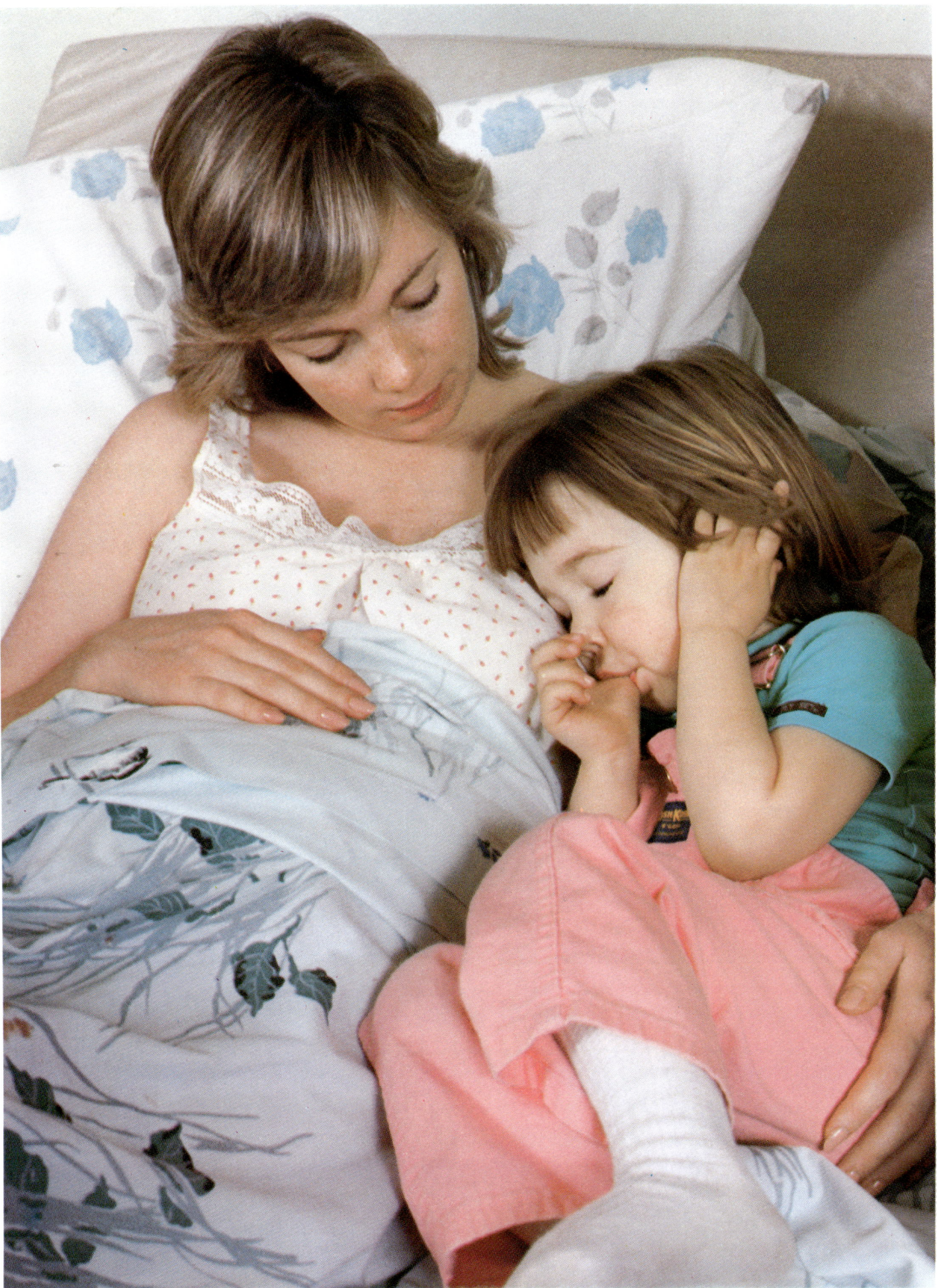

Nancy: I didn't want the day to end. These were the best moments of my life, and I wanted them to last forever.

Tom: Having the extra family members there to share our joy with us made things that much better. Kate's reaction was fun to see. All her giggling and excitement were uncontainable.

Nancy: The birth wouldn't have been as special without Kate there. I just wish she had been a little bit older, because I think her memories of Eric's birth would be much more vivid. I don't know if she'll remember any of the events surrounding his birth, but even if she doesn't, perhaps this experience will help to form some of her later opinions on childbirth.

Birth can and should be a beautiful, loving, miraculous event. It is my hope that Kate's being able to see birth treated in this way will give her a really good feeling about childbirth, and this is something I want to impart to both of my children.

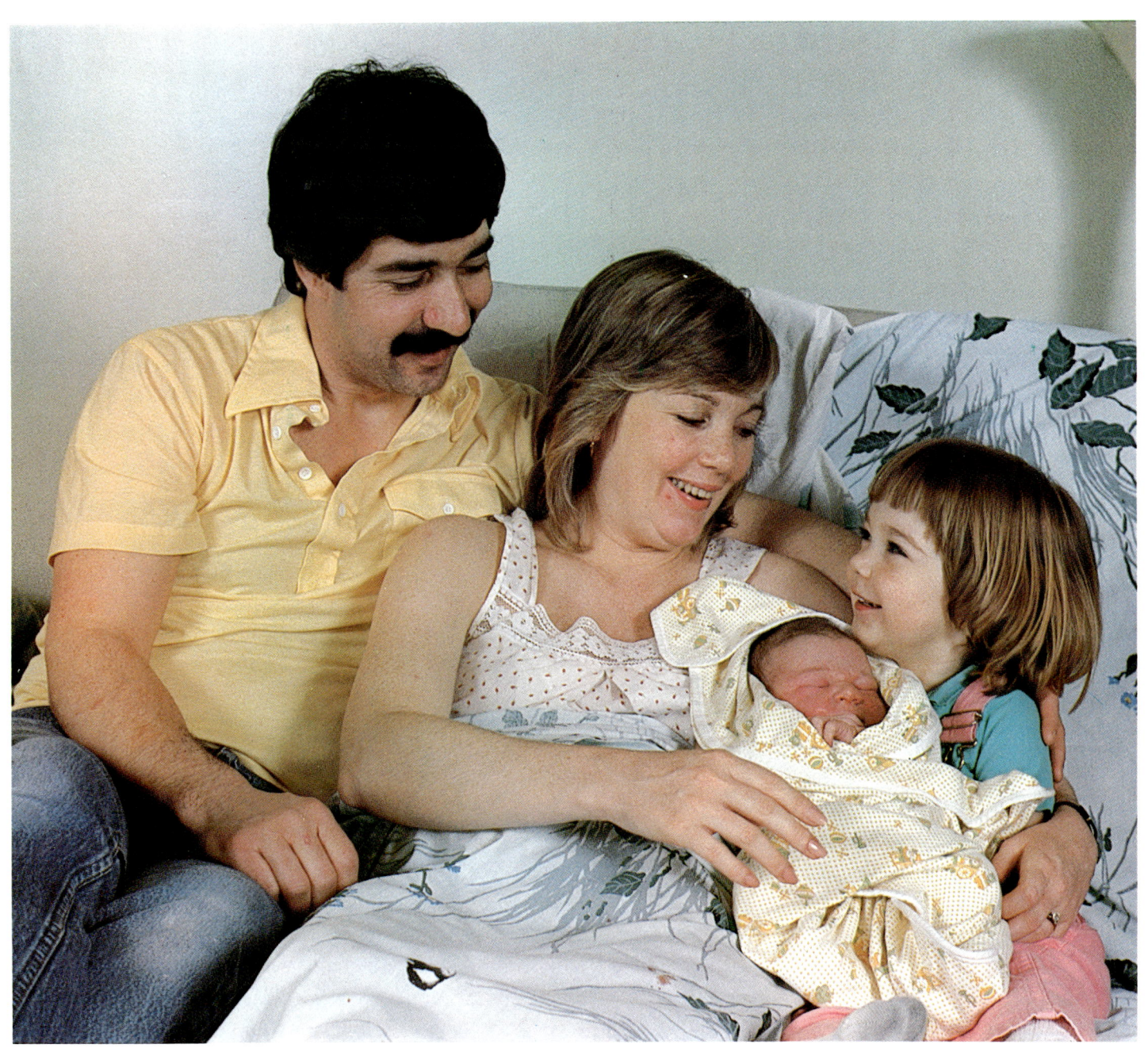

Epilogue

This is the end of our story about Ellen and Ken, Pat and Paul, Susan and David, and Nancy and Tom.

At the same time, it is the beginning of a new chapter in the lives of these four couples. They were active participants in the births of their children by preparing carefully for the event. They knew their options. They had chosen the place where they wanted to give birth, and had chosen to be attended by midwives. Theirs was not a haphazard undertaking, but a well-planned beginning of their children's lives. The couples consciously lived the excitement of the moment, and made the births an all-encompassing experience.

We both feel that we would like these four couples to be models for all who share our belief that childbirth, while sometimes difficult and even painful, is well worth preparing for. Understanding and knowledge of details will help make the birth of one's child a wonderful experience.

Let these moving photographs speak to you and tell you of the deep emotions that these couples felt. We would like them to be an inspiration and guide to you.

KAREN MICHELE
ELISABETH BING